614.518 DOW

DOWDLE, WALTER R.

INFORMED CONSENT

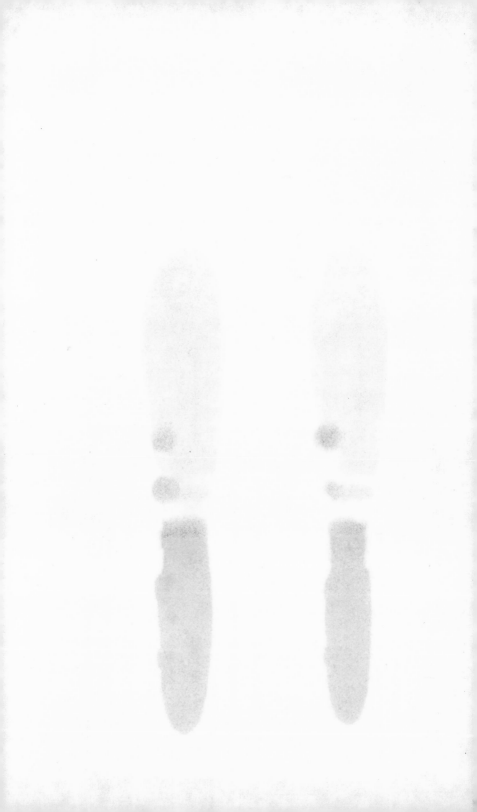

INFORMED CONSENT

INFORMED CONSENT

Influenza Facts and Myths

Walter Dowdle
and Jack LaPatra

NELSON-HALL nh CHICAGO

LIBRARY OF CONGRESS CATALOGING IN PUBLICATION DATA

Dowdle, Walter R.
  Informed consent.

  Includes index.
  1. Influenza.   2. Influenza—Preventative
innoculation.   3. Informed consent (Medical law)
I. LaPatra, Jack W., 1927–   .II. Title.
[DNLM: 1. Informed consent—Popular works.
2. Influenza—Prevention and control—United States
—Popular works.   3. Influenza vaccine—Adverse effects
—Popular works.   4. Public policy—United States—
Popular works.   5. Orthomyxoviruses type A—Popular
works.   WC 515 D45i]
RA644.I6D68   1983   614.5'18   83-4099
ISBN 0-88229-741-4

Manufactured in the United States of America

10 9 8 7 6 5 4 3 2 1

The paper in this book is pH neutral (acid-free).

Contents

Preface

More people are learning about the concept of "informed consent." In spite of implied legalistic formalness, the idea makes a lot of sense. It simply means that before giving consent to undergo any major medical procedure, the patient must be clearly informed in lay terms of the potential benefits and risks of that treatment. The patient should understand what the procedure entails, what alternatives are possible, and what inherent risks of discomfort, serious injury, or death may exist.

Informed consent is not, however, as simple as it may first appear. Many people are highly suggestible. Informing individuals of what might happen can make them believe afterwards that it did happen. When people are given sugar pills (placebo) and told that they may experience relief from symptoms, or side effects such as nausea, dizziness, or sleeplessness, many do. In some instances the very act of soliciting informed consent, if improperly done, may constitute a risk.

The potential adverse effects of suggestive information can be balanced to some degree by telling the patient about the placebo effect and by being specific about the probability of real risk. However, most people are concerned only with effect on themselves, and probability estimates are often difficult to accept. Even though we can accurately predict the statistical effect of an event on a *hypothetical* individual in a population, we can rarely predict the statistical effect of that event on a specific individual. Many people think that the "one in ten thousand could be me." For this reason, as some have pointed out, insurance companies are rich and fortune tellers are poor. These caveats should not detract from the basic right of the American citizen "to know." Our society has assigned the total responsibility for informed consent to the primary medical exam and public health systems. Lost in its concept is that the patient has a responsibility to learn more about the medical procedure he or she will face. Only fully informed people can make intelligent choices.

Formal informed-consent procedures are now used with all vaccines administered in public immunization clinics. Many people first became aware of this practice during the swine flu immunization program of 1976. Before receiving their shots, participants were to read an information statement and to sign registration forms indicating that they understood the benefits and risks of the vaccination. That process was not unlike "preaching to the converted." Few people in those long lines would have been there if they had not already decided to receive the shot. On what "facts" were those individual decisions based?

There is another aspect of informed consent that is rarely mentioned. We give consent through our congressmen and senators to have our tax dollars used for major health initiatives such as the swine flu program of 1976. Regardless of whether one views that program as right or wrong, truly informed consent on such complex issues is difficult. Too often the facts on which to base an intelligent decision are not available. At times it seems as though media figures make such decisions for us. In the case of influenza, the news media have, at best, helped very little. More often they have exploited the sensational aspects of the disease and have been the major sources of erroneous information, which, coupled with the inherent misinformation, myths, and lack of facts regarding influenza, makes informed consent incredibly difficult.

In this book we provide the known facts about the influenza virus and the disease it causes. The history of flu, sometimes called "the last great plague," has the aura and excitement of an epic detective story that has been developing for centuries and is still not solved. We find its story fascinating and hope it will make it easier for each reader to give high-quality informed consent for vaccination against influenza.

CHAPTER 1

The History of a Versatile Virus

Bubonic plague, yellow fever, cholera, typhus, and the classic scourges are generally controlled and restricted to a few geographic areas, but influenza remains unconstrained and misunderstood. Even the architects of our defenses against epidemics, the microbiologists and epidemiologists, admire the ability of the influenza virus to survive.

The average person today has a special connection to influenza. Of the important infectious diseases, flu is the one he or she is almost certain to have experienced during adult life, perhaps several times. Paradoxically, the influenza contact often results in a mild, almost pleasurable episode that offers a few days' vacation from work. Some people have heard of the checkered history of influenza, but to most, it remains almost a joke. In earlier centuries, when typhus, smallpox, typhoid fever, and other killer plagues were present, the sudden appearance of influenza, which, as a rule, killed mostly the old and the weak, was almost a relief.

Studying the history of influenza helps us understand the present and prepare for likely future events. Historical detection of influenza was based not so much on the recorded symptoms of the patients as on the characteristics of the epidemic. Only influenza causes a sudden outbreak of many cases with, after a visit of a few weeks, an almost equally sudden disappearance.

Our knowledge of people's first perceptions of this chameleonlike virus is hazy. Before records were kept, information was passed orally from one generation to the next and distortion of fact occurred. Historians have little doubt that many of the plagues remembered in stories and songs from ancient times were actually influenza epidemics. It is also likely that before the distinctive influenza characteristics became known, other respiratory infections were called flu.

Many believe that the first recorded episode of flu was noted by Diodorus Siculus, who wrote of an epidemic in the Athenian army in Sicily in 415 B.C. Athens mounted an army of five thousand armored men and nearly thirteen hundred archers and slingers. Transported by a hundred-ship armada to Sicily, the army conducted extensive operations; however, they were weakened by an uncertain attitude from Athens, political maneuvering among their officers, and an extended siege at Syracuse. In a climax more exciting than a Hollywood epic, the reinforced Sicilian garrison at Syracuse broke out and pursued the Athenians to the harbor. The Athenians, their equipment in shambles because of the impossibility of long-range maintenance and their ranks decimated by a flu-like illness, were trapped in the harbor, sealed off by a ring of old ships that had been anchored and lashed together. After terrible losses in the harbor, the Athenians fled inland, but the number of sick and dying men increased as their efforts to escape grew more frantic. Those who survived were taken prisoner, packed in concentration camps, and fed on half a slave's ration of meal and water. In eight months most of the prisoners were dead. We can't be sure, but records seem to indicate that the battle-hardened, superior-in-number Athenian soldiers were hurried to defeat by influenza. The short, dry influenza cough was probably as much a sound of the battle scene as the clash of spears and swords.

Athens collapsed in the spring of 404 B.C., and it is likely that the Sicilian tragedy was a significant contributor to the demise of the city-state. The accounts of the events of this period are fragmentary and were first related, not by physicians, but by historians who wanted to impress their readers with tales of the ravages of the disease.

In A.D. 827 an attack of "cough" that spread like a plague was recorded in France. The army of Charlemagne suffered from a flulike illness while returning from Italy in 876. An historian wrote, "Dogs and birds were attacked at this time." In 976 France and Germany were attacked by a fever whose principal symptom was a cough. Influenza may have appeared in England in 996 and 997.

Influenza events may be characterized by a high or low death rate and by a high or low rate of complications. Investigators studying old records often use different criteria to identify the influenza episodes. In the following account, the term *epidemic* connoted local area illness and *pandemic* meant country-wide illness.

Hirsch places the first epidemic that was indisputably influenza in the year 1173; Zeviani in 1293; Gluge in 1323; and Schweich, Biermer, and Ripperger in 1387. In the fourteenth century the Black Death hung like a pall over Europe and Asia. Its characteristic skin hemorrhages wiped out several million people, including an estimated one-quarter of the population of medieval Europe. The plague lasted most of the century and in its wake a weakened mankind fell prey to cholera, typhoid, typhus, smallpox, and certainly influenza. The term *influenza* was first used in 1357. The name for the disease came from the Italian word meaning "influence," since popular belief related the influence of the stars to the appearance of the malady. In spite of the above-mentioned speculations, several other investigators accept nothing prior to the first pandemic of 1510 as being unquestionably influenza.

Flu came and went like a mysterious marauder. Periodic reappearances of influenza were always puzzling. Each new occurrence seemed to be a new illness. In 1485, a flu-like disease called "the sweating sickness" felled hundreds of thousands of Britons. The Royal Navy did not leave port; the lord mayor of London, his successor, and six aldermen died from the fever. Surprisingly, the illness struck down the rich and ignored the poor. A physician wrote of the disease: ". . . when a grete sweyting and stynking, with redness of the face and all of the body, and a contynual thurst, with a grete headache because of the fumes and venoms." Helpless, physicians sat by and waited out the fever, in their frustration prescribing tobacco juice, lime juice, vomiting inducers, and cathartics. Finally, in desperation, the doctors bled their patients. We might suspect that the poor, who could not afford these dubious ministrations, survived because of the lack.

In the sixteenth century some English writers referred to flu as "the new acquaintance." Sir Thomas Randolph, the ambassador of the Court of Queen Elizabeth I to the Court of Mary, Queen of Scots, wrote to Lord Cecil from Edinburgh at the end of November 1562: "May it please your Honor, immediately upon the Quene's [Mary] arivall here, she fell acquainted with a new disease that is common in this towne, called here the newe acquayntance, which passed also throughe her whole courte, neither sparinge lordes, ladies nor damoysells not so much as ether Frenche or English. It ys a plague in their heades that have yt, and a sorenes in their stomackes, with a great coughe, that remayneth with some longer, with others shorter tyme, as yt findeth apte bodies for the nature of the disease. The queen kept her bed six days. There was no appearance of danger, nor manie that die of the disease, excepte some olde folkes."

Most experts agree that an influenza pandemic occurred in 1580. The disease swept out of Asia, spread to Africa and Europe, and then to America in what was possibly the first global spread of the disease. The influenza raged for a month, during which over 90 percent of the population was affected. Then it ended suddenly, as though canceled. Mortality was unusually high due in part, perhaps, to the grisly procedure of bleeding patients with a fever.

In 1658 a famous research physician of London known only as "Dr. Willis" described influenza's calling cards: ". . . a feverish intemperature and whatsoever belongs to this, the heat of the praecordia, thirst, a spontaneous weariness, pain in the head, loyns and limbs, were induced from the blood growing hot and not sufficiently eventilated; hence in many, a part of the thinner blood being heated, and the rest of the liquor being only driven into confusion."

During the period 1700 to 1900 record-keeping improved and historical accounts were plentiful. Many researchers, succumbing to temptation, extrapolated their data back in time and concluded that pandemics have occurred at intervals since ancient times. Obviously, the beginnings of influenza did not coincide with mankind's ability to keep reliable records. Influenza is so ubiquitous and so clinically similar to other illnesses that those who attempted to chronicle it were misled.

The reports of the effects of influenzalike illness include no idea of what agent or condition caused the misery. During the eighteenth and nineteenth centuries, speculation on etiology was lively when the disease was prevalent, but the interest and quality of historical accounts waned during the years between notable outbreaks.

Shortly after the American Revolution, Noah Webster began a scientific investigation of influenza and reported that there had been forty-four appearances of the disease since 1174. He wrote: "The causes most probably exist in the elements, fire, air, and water for we know of no other medium by which diseases can be communicated to whole communities of people." He concluded that influenza was "evidently the effect of some insensible qualities of the atmosphere," an "electric quality."

A hobby among some epidemiologists and virologists is tracing the geographic movements of influenza outbreaks. W. I. B. Beveridge, an authority on influenza, studied the records for the period 1700 to 1900 and concluded that during that time there were seven pandemics and nine other possible pandemics. Beveridge reported that major pandemics took place in 1732–33 and 1781–82. Influenza was worldwide in 1732; there were four minor pandemics in 1742, 1761, 1767, and 1775.

In 1781 a respiratory illness appeared in all European countries and in China, India, and North America. All reports of that period agree that the pandemic started in China in the autumn. Illness rates were high. Thirty thousand people per day were stricken in Leningrad, three-quarters of the residents of Munich fell ill during the winter rampage, and in Rome two-thirds of the population were attacked.

Most experts regard a mild pandemic that occurred in 1788–89 as a recurrence of the 1781–82 event. North America and Europe were affected, but in England the illness was mild and caused hardly any deaths. We might be tempted to pass over this episode as another small wave in the series of waves of illnesses sweeping over mankind. However, we have documentation of the 1789 outbreak of illness as it took place in the United States.

For his dissertation for the degree of doctor of medicine at the University of Pennsylvania in 1793, Robert Johnson studied the influenzalike outbreak of 1789. To orient the reader in time, 1789 was the year Washington was inaugurated as president, the first Congress met in New York, and the French Revolution began. Though the fastest means of travel was horseback, according to Johnson the flu spread like wildfire.

The symptoms of the 1789 illness are described by Johnson as "a sudden onset and four or five days of fever." Recovery was followed by several weeks of persistent coughing and prolonged debility in some cases. People in their middle years were attacked at a high rate. Few died, and Johnson reports that many of the treatments administered were more damaging than simply letting the disease run its course.

Johnson was deeply interested in learning how the disease spread. He was convinced that it passed from person to person by some means, but could not reconcile the contagion mechanism with the speed of propagation that had been recorded. He cited examples from the pandemic of 1782 and noted that infection had appeared in London between May 12 and 18, in Oxford in the third week, and in Edinburgh on May 20. He saw no way that such a rapid spread of disease could be based solely on personal contact.

At another point in his thesis he writes: "On the 2d day of May, 1782, the late Admiral Kempenfelt sailed from Spithead with a squadron under his command, of which the Goliath was one, whose crew was attacked with the influenza, on the 29th of that month: the rest were affected at different times: and so many of the men were rendered incapable of duty by this prevailing sickness, that the whole squadron was obliged to return into port about the second week in June, not having had communication with any shore, and having cruised solely between Brest and the Lizard."

Attempting to explain these mysterious happenings, Johnson writes: "I do not assert, nor do I wish to be understood to mean, that the influenza is not at all contagious: on the contrary, I am possessed of facts which prove in the most incontestable manner, that it may be, and often is propagated from one person to another by means of contagion. But I mean, and the arguments which I have adduced, I trust, will warrant the conclusion that the disease often does arise from some vicious quality of the air, or exhalation in it, as well as from a matter arising from the body of a man labouring under disease." We will never know what Johnson meant by "some vicious quality of the air," but his efforts point out that the infectious disease spread with astonishing speed even before we had fast transportation to blame.

A review of the history of influenza shows that the confusion regarding the origin of the disease manifests itself in a strange way. Everyone assumed that the disease came from somewhere else. In Russia, flu was called the "Chinese disease"; in Germany, the "Russian pest"; the "German disease" in Italy; the "American influenza" in Japan; and in the United States influenza has been known at different times as "Spanish flu" (1918–19), "Asian flu" (1957–58), "Hong Kong flu" (1968–69), "London flu" (1972–73), "Russian flu" (1977–78), and "Brazilian flu" (1978–79).

In 1889 a major pandemic was recorded. It was named the "Asiatic influenza pandemic," and its itinerary would be attractive to the most seasoned world traveler. The disease departed Bukhara in Russia in May and after a leisurely excursion reached Tomsk and the Caucasus in October. The flu reached North America in December, paused in South America between February and April, and in the spring arrived in India and Australia. A high attack rate brought many deaths.

The pandemic was relatively mild in America. Some doctors labeled it "Chinese distemper" and maintained that the disease's origin was in the dust eddying from the parched banks of the Yellow River. Another group of physicians called the disease "Russian influenza."

The 1889 pandemic is historically important in two

ways. First, prior to this pandemic, the eminent British epidemiologist, Charles Creighton, asserted that influenza was not spread by contagion. Data from epidemics showed that most parts of a large country were affected within two or three weeks, a large population within a considerable radius almost at once, and the occupants of the same house simultaneously. Surely, this couldn't be contagion.

Pasteur's work had convinced most doctors that germs were the cause of infectious diseases. With such great emphasis on finding a bacterial cause, a presumed bacterial cause was found. In Germany, Richard Pfeiffer discovered a particular bacterium present in great numbers in the throats of influenza victims. The bacterium did not appear in persons unless they had recently recovered from influenza. The bacterium was also associated with the lesions of the disease. For the first time in history a majority of medical people believed the cause of influenza had been discovered. The second important aspect of the 1889 pandemic is the belief that it was the predecessor of the most serious pandemic of all times in 1918–19. The 1889 experience was a warning—but there was no one listening.

The social and medical importance of the 1918–19 influenza pandemic cannot be overemphasized. It is generally believed that about half of the 2 billion people living on earth in 1918 became infected with flu. Some 22 million persons died. In the United States, 20 million flu cases were counted and about half a million people died. It is impossible to imagine the social misery and dislocation implicit in these dry statistics.

The 1918 pandemic is cited as the most graphic display ever of the potential biological muscle of influenza. The world has never been quite the same since that event. Historians place it with the other major human catastrophes— the plague of Justinian, bubonic plague, which killed several million people in Byzantium in A.D. 542; and the carnage of the Black Death, also bubonic plague, which killed about 25 million people in Europe during the middle ages.

Three interrelated waves made up the massive pandemic. The first began in April 1918 in France, then spread to the rest of Europe and the United States. India and New Zealand were struck in July, and in August the virus hit South Africa. The second wave in the fall of 1918 involved nearly every nation in the world. The third wave swept over Great Britain and the United States in February and March 1919. Only the tiny island of Tristan da Cunha, isolated in the South Atlantic, escaped untouched. Even remote, inaccessible Inuit villages were discovered with every resident dead.

The overall 1918–19 pandemic experience was unique. The rates of incidence of disease and subsequent death were incredibly high. Had the pandemic continued at its accelerating rate, mankind would have suffered immeasurable damage in a few weeks. By some unknown mechanism, the pandemic began, spread, and then abruptly stopped, leaving a traumatized world to go about its business.

In contrast to the past, many cases and deaths occurred among young adults, not just the very young and very old as before. In the first wave the number of cases often exceeded 50 percent of the total population, but the number of deaths was low. The second wave was lethal, and in as many as 80 percent of all the attacks a different manifestation of the disease appeared. Two not previously seen forms of infection were observed. In the first, the illness began with acute inflammation of the lungs, resulting in excessive fluid in the lung tissues, discoloration of the mucous membranes, and death within a few days. The second form of infection developed into bronchopneumonia on the fourth or fifth day, which was followed either by death or a long convalescence.

Of special interest to us are the events in the United States in 1918. The country had mounted an army of 2 million men, ten times the peacetime level, and was fighting World War I. The army was fueled by a flow of country boys from rural America, who moved through hastily thrown-up camps onto jammed troop ships to cross the Atlantic and then settled into a dangerous, debilitating life in the trenches. In those early months of 1918, scant attention was paid to an epidemic of "grippe." After all, there had been mild epidemics in both 1915 and 1916.

An examination of the 1918 volumes of the *Journal of the American Medical Association* does not reveal a mention of the spring epidemic. Routine reporting of incidences of influenza did not exist in those days. Deaths were recorded and pneumonia was usually given as cause of death in cases of respiratory illness. Most citizens, and many doctors, couldn't tell a cold from the flu, and bacteriological tests weren't helpful. There was no tightly woven network of federal, state, and local public health departments to put together what data did exist to give a sketch of the epidemic. The only significant records we have from 1918 are from organizations and institutions, such as the army and prisons, that had complete jurisdiction over their members.

The clues were there, that spring of 1918, but it was only much later that statisticians discovered that an unanticipated number of people had died of respiratory illness during the early months of 1918. In the few postmortems of that period something new was observed about the lungs of the victims, and, unlike any previous epidemic, young adults were being struck by the infection. With our eyes and energies on the war, not even the mystery, much less the solution, was discovered. Crosby, writing in 1975, sets the scene for us: "The United States was not merely unprepared to control the spread of influenza. It had carefully, if unintentionally, prepared itself to expedite the cultivation and dissemination of just precisely the influenza virus of Fall 1918. Among adult males, those who were most susceptible to the Spanish influenza were men of military age. They were also the most susceptible to secondary complications, such as pneumonia.''

''So at the end of the last summer of World War I some 1.5 million American adults who were most perfectly qualified to cultivate the most dangerously virulent strain of influenza virus in history and its jackal bacteria were living cheek-by-jowl in a small number of military camps all over the nation, and large numbers of them were constantly traveling back and forth between these camps. All that was needed was the proper germ.''

In the midst of the chaos of the pandemic that followed, epidemiologists and scientists were hard at work. It was their opportunity to take grim advantage of the presence of this elusive disease. In spite of earlier observations and conclusions to the contrary, the speed at which the infection spread was accounted for by the speed of available transportation and in many instances by the arrival of infected individuals.

The evidence of speed of spread, however, was not conclusive. Strange skips in infected populations occurred. For example, Boston and Bombay had their epidemic peaks in the same week, while in New York, only a few hours away from Boston by train, the peak came three weeks later. The transportation theory substantiated the spread of the disease over long distances more easily than over short distances in some cases.

It seemed obvious that more than one dissemination mechanism was operating in the 1918 pandemic. The most common speculation among scientists was that widespread disposition of some impotent form of the cause of infection happened at an earlier time. Only a trigger—one that affected wide geographic areas—was required to set the pandemic in motion. But there was not a shred of evidence to support this idea.

Many efforts were made to prove contagiousness—some contrived and some natural. In one contagion experiment, sixty-two volunteers between fifteen and thirty-four years of age were used. Samples of secretions from the noses and throats of infected patients were sprayed in the same areas of the volunteers. Nothing happened. In another experiment, acutely ill patients breathed and coughed into the faces of volunteers. Again, nothing happened. The transmission of the sickness from person to person was not demonstrated in the laboratory. With the benefit of hindsight, we suspect now that what was being tested was the immunity of the volunteers. It's very likely that the volunteers had had a previous minor experience with the infection, perhaps even without being aware of it.

The efforts to confirm the Pfeiffer bacterium as the causal agent of influenza were confusing and contradictory. It is technically very difficult to isolate this organism from the respiratory tract. But the failure to prove or disprove the etiological relationship between the Pfeiffer bacterium and flu had a positive payoff. Instinctively, researchers were beginning to suspect that a virus was the cause.

Scientists made an enormous effort to determine the cause of influenza during the 1918 pandemic. Discrediting earlier theories cannot be called success, but during this frenetic activity, something took place that offered fresh new clues to the cause of influenza. While the human race was in agony at the height of the second wave of the 1918 pandemic, a new disease appeared among swine in the Middle West. Thousands of swine died, and millions fell ill. Was this just a coincidence? Dr. J. S. Koen, an inspector in the Division of Hog Cholera Control of the United States Bureau of Animal Industry, didn't think so. He was sure the disease hadn't been seen before in swine, and he was so taken by the resemblance of the signs and symptoms seen in man to those observed in the swine that he called the new disease "swine flu."

Koen's speculation about a connection between the influenza pandemic and the swine epizootic (animal epidemic) was not popular. People who enjoyed eating pork or who made their living in the pork industry feared the impact of public knowledge that swine could acquire human influenza.

Koen stuck by his evidence, saying that "the similarity of the epidemic among people and the epizootic among pigs was so close, the reports so frequent, that an outbreak in the family would be followed immediately by an outbreak among the hogs, and vice versa, as to present a most striking coincidence, if not suggesting a close relation between the two conditions. It looked like 'flu', and until proved it was not 'flu', I shall stand by that diagnosis."

A major breakthrough came in 1928 through the efforts of G. N. McBryde and veterinarians of the Bureau of Animal Industry. They successfully transmitted the infection from pig to pig by taking mucus from the respiratory tract of sick pigs and placing it in the noses of healthy pigs. When they filtered the mucus before transferring it, the pigs rarely got sick.

The development of bacterial filters plays an important part in this story. The filters used in 1918 made it clear that some diseases are caused by microbes smaller than bacteria. These microbes were called "filterable" viruses, because they penetrated filters that stopped bacteria, or "ultra-visible" viruses, because they could not be seen with the ordinary microscope. Now we call these microbes viruses. The notion that influenza was caused by a virus could not be verified during and after the 1918 pandemic because of unreliable filters.

The role of the Pfeiffer bacillus remained a mystery through this period. Although there was no trace of the bacillus in the lungs of some 1918 pandemic victims, it was present in the lungs of many others. But often the bacillus was not found when an autopsy was conducted.

The tiny, delicate, and hard-to-detect bacillus was thought by some to disintegrate at the patient's death. Others, like Dr. Emile Roux, director of the Pasteur Institute in Paris during the 1918 pandemic, theorized that the bacillus was only a fellow traveler and not the culprit. Under the direction of Dr. Roux, a series of experiments had been conducted that convinced him that Pfeiffer's bacillus was not the cause of the infection, and neither was any other bacterium—not the streptococcus, or the pneumococcus, or the staphylococcus. Nearly a decade passed after Dr. Roux's experiments and Dr. Koen's speculations before the last ingredient—a technological development—enabled the next step toward an understanding of influenza.

In 1928 Dr. Richard Shope, a pathologist with the Rockefeller Institute, began an intensive study of swine flu. At that time the institute was dedicated to the proposition that many of the basic phenomena of human disease can best be studied in animals and plants. Shope, a brilliant and unconventional thinker, was intrigued by Koen's efforts of a decade earlier. He visited pig farmers in the Midwest, where he found that swine flu still appeared every fall.

Using much-improved filters, he repeated earlier experiments and showed that after bacteria had been removed, the disease could still be transferred repeatedly in pigs. Shope's work was the first reliable experimental evidence that influenza is caused by a virus. The gate that was opened by this research allowed further research along these lines that contributed to the understanding of influenza in man.

Shope also found that the virus that caused influenza works with a cohort, a bacterium that is a hog variant of

Pfeiffer's bacillus. Apparently this bacterium, though not the cause of flu, increases the severity of the infection. From the foundation of this animal research, it was easy to infer that when Pfeiffer's bacillus and the flu virus occur together in man, a severe and often fatal pneumonia results.

Shope's milestone work in 1931 gave a first peek at the complex etiology of influenza. The virus, which neither he nor anyone else actually saw, was detected as a causal agent by the observation of its effect—the disease influenza. And that causal link could not be verified unless all other possible causes were removed. The complex technical processes using bacteria filters made this possible.

An apparent epidemic of influenza struck England and Wales in December 1932. Three scientists, Wilson Smith, Patrick Laidlaw, and Christopher Andrewes, were studying viruses at the National Institute for Medical Research in London at the time. The institute decided to make an effort to find the cause of the epidemic. The researchers set to work, following a strategy of injecting filtered material from human throat samples into various laboratory animals.

A critical ingredient of this research was adapted from the work of Shope. Animals struggled violently when drops from throat samples were put in their noses, and often a sneeze would hurl a lethal dose back at the scientist. To avoid this, animals were anesthetized. With this technique, the animals got not only a primary infection but also pneumonia, just like people. It was clear that while an animal was anesthetized, fluids inserted into the nose went all the way to the lungs. A simulation of the actual process was accomplished. Research proceeded briskly, and although still no one had seen the virus, the presumed cause of influenza was identified and isolated.

In addition to achieving those marvelous results, Smith, Laidlaw, and Andrewes demonstrated that mice, if they survived the infection and the accompanying pneumonia, became immune to reinfection. The scientists identified the proteins (antibodies) that fought the virus. The name "WS" was given to the virus isolated by the team in honor of their leader, Wilson Smith. Dr. Thomas Francis, Jr., a scientist working in Puerto Rico in 1934 under the auspices of the Rockefeller Foundation, made the second isolate of a virus. It was dubbed "PR/8."

Wilson Smith added to the knowledge about flu by discovering in 1935 that influenza virus can be grown in fertile hens' eggs. Up to 10 billion viruses were harvested after two days of incubation. The ease with which the influenza virus was produced attracted the attention of virologists around the world. As a result we now know more about this virus than any other that affects man.

A consequence of Smith's flu virus production technique was the possibility of a vaccine. Beginning in 1936 and continuing to the end of the decade, vaccines containing both live and dead viruses were tested. When people were vaccinated with these test vaccines, antibodies to the virus appeared, but rarely in numbers sufficient to protect the people from the infection.

In 1940 Francis and Magill isolated an influenza virus strain different from WS and PR/8. They named it the "Lee" strain. Eventually it was learned that there are at least three different types of the flu virus, all of which have the same appearance under the electron microscope. The types were simplistically designated A, B, and C.

In the late forties, a virus nomenclature scheme was adopted that identified the type and family of the virus, the place it was isolated, its identifying number, the year of isolation, and some of its chemical aspects. To date, thousands of strains of A virus have been listed.

The decade of the thirties produced much knowledge about viruses, but the fear of a repeat of the 1918 pandemic was as strong as ever. Efforts to produce a successful vaccine were relentless. The basic problem was balancing the vaccine strength against its side effects. To produce enough antibodies to protect from infection required a vaccine strength that gave side effects as uncomfortable as the infection itself.

In 1941, Francis and Salk produced a successful vaccine consisting of two strains of influenza A virus and one of B. The vaccine gave protection against the viruses of that time for about one year.

In 1947 recently vaccinated people began getting the flu. Researchers found that the A strain had changed and a new vaccine was required. Eventually scientists speculated that new types of viruses emerged periodically and that variants of these types appeared every few years. These changes must be monitored and anticipated in order to provide effective vaccines. The influenza virus is versatile.

Efforts to track down remnants of the 1918 pandemic continued. In an exciting piece of detective work, scientists learned that an army transport ship sailed from Seattle to Nome in November 1918 during the height of the influenza attack. Infection spread throughout the ship on the voyage. In Nome the very ill were nursed by Inuit women, and many Inuit perished in the subsequent epidemic. They and many of their infectors were buried in the frozen earth of Alaska.

In 1951, after this information became known, concern developed that the vicious virus of the 1918 pandemic was dormant, but alive, in the permafrost of Alaska. So deep was the concern that a team of scientists went to that frozen land and exhumed several well-preserved Inuit bodies buried in the tundra at Golovin. Samples of lung tissue were tested using ferrets, just as Wilson Smith and his colleagues had done nineteen years before. The tests showed no sign of viral activity. Apparently the virus perished in the icy grave.

Had the Spanish influenza strain disappeared? No one knew the answer to this question. Dr. Andrewes, the only surviving member of the team that had isolated the influenza virus, commented: "Most people believe it [the virus] goes, metaphorically speaking, 'underground.' It is rarely recovered from flu-like illnesses between epidemics. There is a strong suggestion, however, that it can persist in an area without causing outbreaks. . . . I can believe that the virus goes underground and perhaps does so all over the world, causing odd subclinical infections and not much more, but able to become active and epidemic when the time is ripe. . . . We cannot, unfortunately, say that influenza is yet a certainly preventable disease and it is still possible that a pandemic might return and kill its millions, as happened in 1918–19."

On this topic, Sir Frank MacFarlane Burnet, a leading Australian microbiologist, said in 1952: "Of all the virus diseases, influenza is probably that in which mutational changes in the virus are of greatest human importance. We can only guess what type of virus was responsible in 1918–19 and what changes took place during the course of the pandemic. But even in the period since the human virus was first isolated in 1933 there have been striking changes in the immunological character of both influenza A and B viruses. Some of us believe that the influenza virus' chief means of survival is its capacity for constant mutation to new serological patterns, and those of us who have had anything to do with the production of influenza vaccines know very well how that capacity can nullify the most painstaking work."

Somewhere in mainland China (perhaps western Kweichow and eastern Yunnain) the next pandemic started in 1957. The "Asian" flu erupted in February and reached Europe and America in June. The following winter, the attack rate was 50 to 70 percent for the ten- to twenty-year-old age group, 20 to 40 percent for those between the ages

of twenty and fifty years, and it was even lower for older
people. Nearly 70,000 deaths, mostly people over sixty-
five, were attributed to the infection in the United States
during the winter of 1957–58. Ten years later, in July
1968, a new strain called the "Hong Kong" virus began in
southeast China. That winter over 30,000 people died in
the United States.

In January 1976 there was an apparent outbreak of swine
flu at Fort Dix, New Jersey. Concern swept through the
medical and scientific community. Perhaps the Spanish
flu had returned and a repeat of the 1918 pandemic was
imminent. A complex vaccination program was mounted,
but the "Spanish lady" did not appear that year.

Ironically, in just the following year, an earlier epidemic virus did reappear. As it turned out, it was not the
virus of 1918 but a virus which had been prevalent during
the mid-fifties and had not been isolated since 1956. Like
its previous pandemic strains the Russian flu virus seems
to have caused outbreaks in China before appearing in the
Soviet Union in the fall of 1977. Unlike its previous pandemic strains this virus did not cause large numbers of
deaths, primarily because all older persons, or anyone
born before 1957, were already immune. The 1977 Russian flu virus spread rapidly throughout the world causing
outbreaks in schools and other institutions with populations which had been born after 1957. Where did the virus
actually come from? Where had it been since 1956?

From 1977 until the present, two distinct type A viruses
and their variants have caused outbreaks, epidemics, and
deaths, a phenomenon unprecedented in the modern history of influenza.

What can be learned from the history of influenza? Perhaps little from the early chronicle of the disease with its
folklore, imprecise description, and confusions of medical terms. However, since the advent of modern virology
in 1933, we have learned enough about the variability of

the virus and its potential for epidemic disease so that we cannot dismiss some of the earlier accounts. The virus of influenza is highly versatile.

To identify some of the questions we can't answer, let us choose a well-documented event in the history of influenza—the 1918–19 pandemic. For example, influenza is almost always a mild illness, causing death mostly among the aged and infirm. If this is so, how can the 1918–19 carnage be called flu at all? Though the epidemic spread like wildfire—like flu, unlike any other known viral epidemic—it killed too many people and in the wrong age ranges.

Perhaps the war exacerbated the pandemic. Possibly poverty and poor diet and sanitation contributed; or maybe the massive movement of troops and shifting of civilian populations were involved. But the disease also struck quiet, rural communities.

Why did pneumonia, usually the executioner of the old, prefer young adults in 1918–19? In effect, the events of that year could be called a pandemic of pneumonia. How could pneumonia, caused by bacteria like strep and staph, change simultaneously into vicious strains of organisms that behaved differently?

One theory about Spanish flu suggests that two (or more) organisms cooperated to create a unique disease. This is just a conjecture, and the problems of testing it in the laboratory have been likened to "juggling eggs and cannon balls together with precision and grace."

When autopsies of victims of the fall wave were done, the lungs were brimming with thin, bloody fluid, and some were completely free of bacteria. This meant that the invading organism had spread over the vast expanses of the lining of the respiratory apparatus before the body could mobilize its defenses. How could this happen? Why did the 1957 pandemic, like the one in 1889 and unlike the one in 1918, kill few people? Even after enormous advances in the science of virology we don't know the answer.

Our inability to understand influenza events of this century is the best evidence of the uncertainty associated with an "history of influenza." We have no complete virological history of flu before 1933. The history of influenza virus was summarized in one sentence by Charles Cockburn in 1973. As head of the virus section of the World Health Organization, Cockburn said: "The influenza virus behaves just as it seems to have done five hundred or one thousand years ago, and we are no more capable of stopping epidemics or pandemics than our ancestors were."

CHAPTER 2

Getting to Know the Flu Virus

Science is simple—it's the vocabulary that's difficult! For most people, scientific pronouncements are overwhelming. New words are being added almost daily, and the meanings of old words often change as new information is uncovered. But like all words, scientific terms are simply ways of conveying complex combinations of thoughts in shorthand.

It is ironic that the words essential to scientific progress are often the major obstacles to the exchange of meaningful messages between the scientists and the general public. Just as in learning a foreign language, however, knowing a few words can prove to be immensely valuable. In this book, we keep the technical jargon to a minimum. But some words cannot be avoided. If you don't have some background in biology, spend a little time on the next few pages to learn the language. Through it you can share with us an awareness of an interesting part of our world—the virus.

First we introduce the three influenza virus "families"—A, B, and C. We know a lot about virus A, less about B, and little about C. Since C causes only mild respiratory illness, less attention has been paid to it. However, we do know that C is more different from A and B than the latter two are from each other. Let's take a careful look at influenza virus A, recognizing that most of the facts apply also to B.

As viruses go, the influenza virus is medium sized, about four-millionths of an inch in diameter. It is five times larger than the polio virus and three times smaller than the smallpox virus. The shape of the complete particle may vary from round to elongated. The virus presents a strange face to the world. Its surface is studded with spikes composed of protein containing a small amount of complex sugars. Most of the spikes, called *hemagglutinins*, have a sharp tip and are triangular in cross section. They have the special ability to cause red blood cells to clump. We cannot see the virus in a test tube, but if red blood cells of many animals, including man, chickens, and guinea pigs, are added and they stick together, we know the virus is there.

The rest of the spikes look like small mushrooms and are named *neuraminidase*. These blunt spikes contain an *enzyme* which acts on a complex sugar found on the surface of most living cells to release *neuraminic* acid.

The bases of the spikes are embedded in a thin layer of *lipid*, a fatlike substance on the surface of the virus. The lipid surrounds a protein matrix, or superstructure, which gives the virus its shape. The matrix, in turn, houses and protects the viral genetic material *ribonucleoprotein* (RNA) and the three enzymes needed to assist in replication. The virus is like a free-floating spaceship with the hundreds of spikes acting as multiple landing gear. The lipid layer is the tough protective skin; the protein matrix forms the structural walls; the RNA is the computer information center; and the internal enzymes supply the tools needed for building other spaceships should the proper factory be found.

If the viral spaceship causes infection in an animal that survives, within two or three weeks large quantities of *antibodies* appear in the fluid portion of the blood of the survivor. These antibodies are one of the body's primary defenses against foreign substances, called *antigens*. In the case of the virus, the body recognizes that the hemagglutinin, the neuraminidase, the matrix protein, and the ribonucleoprotein are foreign. Consequently, antibodies mounted against these invaders can be used as tools for identifying and characterizing influenza viruses. A serum containing antibodies prepared for this purpose is called an *antiserum*. Antiserums against the matrix protein or ribonucleoprotein can be used to identify a virus as *type A, B,* or *C*. We can use antiserums against the surface spike proteins to identify the virus as to *subtype* and even to *strain*, thereby providing the basis for the current influenza virus nomenclature that seems to be a never-ending source of confusion to the news media and the public. But influenza virus nomenclature is simple too, once the rules are known. After a virus is isolated in a laboratory and shown to be an influenza virus type A, B, or C, it is given a name according to the rules of international nomenclature established by the World Health Organization (WHO). For example, virus isolate number 32 from an influenza A outbreak in Hong Kong in 1982 would be designated: A/Hong Kong/32/82.

This doesn't, however, give us any information about the antigenic characteristics of the hemagglutinin (H) or the neuraminidase (N) surface antigens, both of which provide important epidemiologic and biologic information. To bring some order out of the chaos created by the constant mutations of the H and N antigens and the vast array of antigens found among other mammals and birds, WHO has established a bank of reference antisera covering distinct groupings of H and N antigens. For example, influenza type A viruses isolated from humans during the period from 1933 to 1956 all fall into the grouping of H1N1. Those from 1957 to 1967 can be grouped into the subtypes H2N2. From 1968 to the present they are designated H3N2, since only the H antigens changed. Therefore, the complete name would be: A/Hong Kong/32/82(H3N2).

Enormous variation within the designated groupings still exists. This is usually resolved by selecting one or more epidemiologically important strains as WHO reference strains. In more recent times, for example, the news media have referred to the "Victoria" flu or the "Texas" flu. These are all H3N2 strains, but they represent significant antigenic variation from the parent 1968 strains.

At some time in our lives we learned the difference between a boulder and a tree, a sculpture of a kitten and a real kitten, a salt crystal and a bacterium. The second one in each pair has the ability to absorb nutrients, convert them into essential body materials, and grow through the process of cell division. The growing tips of the tree are rapidly dividing cells that become leaves, outer and inner bark, cambium, and wood. The kitten grows in the same way, with rapidly dividing cells forming even more complex organs. The bacteria, for the most part, remain as single cells, but the bacterial cell can grow into a culture by dividing, just as the cells that compose more complex living things do. A virus doesn't grow at all. It replicates.

A few years ago it was fashionable for biologists to ask whether a virus was "living" or "nonliving." In the world outside the cell, the virus is not capable of absorbing nutrients and is certainly not able to divide. In this respect it is like the salt crystal—nonliving. Even more like salt, some viruses may form crystals when in pure form. But once the virus is inside a plant or animal cell, offspring appear by the thousands in short order.

Some bacteria, such as rickettsia, the cause of Rocky Mountain spotted fever, grow like a virus in a living cell, but in the cell the bacteria never lose their identity. They always look like bacteria. Not the virus. Once it enters a cell it cannot be found. When bacteria are in the cell they multiply by cell division, like any other of their kind. The virus uses the cell's metabolic machinery to create exact copies of itself. None of this fits our concept of a living thing, but that is *our* shortcoming. On any given hour of a day there are far more virus particles being formed than people. It matters little that this method of reproduction doesn't fit into our scheme of things. The virus is a highly successful member of our living world.

Here is how virus reproduction takes place. When the virus lands on a cell, the triangular spikes attach to the neuraminic acid molecule described earlier. If the virus makes a poor choice and sticks to a nonliving substance or a nonsusceptible cell, the enzyme of the blunt spikes leaps into action, dissolving the bond between the neuraminic acid and the sharp spikes. The virus springs free, ready to try its luck elsewhere. If the virus happens to find a susceptible cell, there are two ways the virus might enter. In the first strategy, the target cell sends out short "feelers" which surround the virus and form a little sac. Unaware of the consequences of its action, the cell absorbs the sac in a *vacuole,* which is gradually assimilated into the cell *cytoplasm.* This normal response of cells to many small foreign objects is just what the virus wants. The second ploy the attached influenza virus might use to enter the target cell is to blend the virus membrane with the cell membrane. In either case, once inside the cell, the virus disintegrates in minutes to release its vital parts into the cytoplasm. The process of using the cell to supply building materials for more virus particles begins immediately.

The virus releases into the host cell eight separate pieces of RNA, or genes. These give information for the building blocks and helper substances needed to make more virus particles. The virus also supplies three enzymes that use the information to manufacture pieces of RNA that are mirror images of those released into the cell. The mirror images become the patterns from which the cell builds each of its virus parts.

As the virus parts appear in the cell fluid, they begin to migrate to the cell surfaces. The sticky ends of the spikes become embedded in the cell's own surface membrane, and the matrix protein, like so many bricks, falls into place under the membrane. An arch is formed, under which the genetic information and essential internal enzymes begin to assemble. We don't know how the eight separate pieces of RNA get together, but the matrix bricks continue to fall into place, bulging from the cell surface until a closed sphere or tube is formed.

At the same time, the neuraminidase, the enzyme spike on the surface of the newly created virus, is destroying all the neuraminic acid it can find on the virus surface or on the cell membrane. Without this mopping-up exercise, the newly formed virus particles would stick to each other or to the cell, and go nowhere. Thanks to the neuraminidase, the new virus particles release, ready to move on and begin a life of their own.

In this way the cell forms thousands of virus particles that bud continuously from the surface for hours and sometimes days, until finally the cell dies from exhaustion. The released viruses infect and kill other cells, and the cycle continues. A viral birth is a simple but highly sophisticated means for self-replication that works very well.

Schoolchildren study the butterfly, whose eggs produce caterpillars that spin webs, eat leaves, form cocoons and develop into butterflies that repeat the cycle. The time and energy expended in this process is enormous. Biologically, living things have only one purpose—to reproduce. Everything else is extraneous. The influenza virus cuts the extraneous activity to a minimum. Other viruses have even more efficient methods for perpetuating themselves. Although the lifestyle of the influenza virus doesn't seem like much fun, you must admit that it focuses on its basic purpose and accomplishes it in a no-nonsense fashion.

Ego, which seems reserved to humans, makes us think of viruses and the diseases they cause in terms of ourselves and extensions of ourselves, such as our livestock, crops, and pets. But when we look carefully, we find that most living creatures have their own virus problems. We are not alone. We may get some perverse satisfaction from the knowledge that the same bacteria that can infect us with typhoid or cholera can themselves be infected by their own special viruses.

What is the source of all these viruses? How long have they existed? We can't be sure. Since viruses leave no fossils, we are left to our own ingenuity in answering these questions. For many years we thought that viruses might be descendants of larger, more complex disease organisms. Another popular theory portrayed viruses as the descendants of primitive, precellular forms of life that survived only in the sheltered environment of the cells of higher organisms. The first idea fails to explain the source of viruses because none of the known viruses have any features remotely resembling the cellular organization of other disease-producing agents. The second theory doesn't explain how life forms more primitive than viruses existed in the absence of a living cell.

The electron microscope allows us to recognize structural patterns common to viruses in the animal and plant kingdoms. Many of these configurations housing the virus genetic material resemble certain organelles, such as microtubules and filaments found in plant and animal cells, and, like the virus, are formed through self-assembly of simple repeating protein building blocks. Perhaps viruses are renegade cellular elements that went off on their own. But total independence remains elusive; the virus must return to the cell to replicate.

Viruses are part of an extended family. Over thirty groups of viruses infect plants and animals. Some viruses have geometric structures with twenty sides, but differ in the number and size of their protein building blocks. Some viruses are tubular, others are spherical or elongated and are covered with a thin membrane. A few are bullet shaped, and some viruses of bacteria resemble tadpoles. The basic structures of all viruses are formed according to the physical laws of crystals. Many viruses may have crossed the barrier between plants and animals, and certainly others have crossed species barriers within the plant and animal kingdoms. Some viruses, such as those that cause yellow fever and certain forms of encephalitis, replicate in mammals, mosquitoes, and birds. Other viruses cause only minor disease in their preferred hosts, such as the Lassa fever virus in rodents, but severe infections in man. Other viruses are very fussy about the species they will infect.

Influenza A viruses are also found in birds, pigs, and horses. Even cattle and dogs are sometimes infected by A viruses. Many influenza viruses live in harmony with certain water bird species, suggesting that the influenza viruses originated with birds. No influenza B viruses have been found in birds or, indeed, in any other animal except man.

An influenza A virus was first isolated in 1901 from chickens during a fowl plague epidemic in Italy. This lethal disease of chickens surfaced in Italy in 1878 and later in other European countries. The disease was not like influenza and the agent was not suspected of belonging to the influenza family of viruses until modern laboratory methods of analysis were used in 1955. A little later, influenza viruses were recognized in ducks in England and in

Czechoslovakia. In the 1970s, viruses were discovered in a wide variety of domestic and wild bird species, including chickens, terns, quail, turkeys, puffins, parrots, cockatoos, parakeets, shearwaters, ducks of all species, myna birds, finches, hornbills, tanagers, and orioles.

Influenza virus infections either kill birds or affect them not at all. Some viruses in chickens, turkeys, and terns cause death. Some viral strains cause a respiratory disease in domestic ducks and quail. Viruses in turkeys may cause a drop in egg production, but no obvious disease.

Influenza viruses cause infections in many young migratory birds, arctic terns, ducks, puffins, and shearwaters, and large numbers of virus particles are shed without any signs of disease. These birds might trigger epidemics among domestic fowl by contaminating the water courses along the natural flyways. During cold weather, the viruses may remain in the water in an infectious state for weeks. Contaminated water is probably the major factor in the transmission of influenza viruses in nature.

In 1918 pigs suffered from minor epidemics of influenza when the great pandemic struck the human population. Whether influenza in pigs occurred before that time we cannot be sure, although there were earlier reports. The influenza virus that was first recovered from pigs in 1930 was later shown to be closely related to the virus occurring in man in about 1918 to 1929. Pig populations celebrate influenza annually, much like their human cousins. The rarely fatal disease in pigs resembles influenza in humans, and farmers merely ignore it. The viruses causing outbreaks in pigs have not changed much since 1930. We call the disease "classical" swine influenza. Disease caused by these viruses is common in North America and has been reported in Hong Kong, Taiwan, Italy, and Japan—all trading partners of the United States. While pigs don't fly south for the winter, the new piglets that appear in the herds annually and breeding stock that is shipped every-

where keep the virus going. Pigs are also infected with the
influenza viruses of man. Since 1968 each new human influenza variant has found its way into the pig population,
where it may cause widespread infection but little disease.

Historians insist that horses have suffered in human influenza epidemics, but we have no proof. The first influenza virus from horses was isolated in 1956 in Czechoslovakia. This subtype remained the only known virus of
horses until 1963, when a new influenza A virus subtype
outbreak occurred among the most pampered horses in the
world, race horses in Miami. This new subtype spread rapidly among horses around the world. The virus appeared
mysteriously, and observers noted that its surface antigens
closely resembled influenza viruses isolated from ducks in
the Ukraine that same year. Don't ask how that happened.

Both the 1956 and the 1963 subtype continue to cause
influenza in race horses. Though rarely fatal, the illness
causes complicated economic losses since race horses are
the principal victims. With race horses, as with pigs, the
disease is kept in circulation through the annual introduction of new unprotected hosts and by the movement of infected animals. There is no evidence that horses are infected with influenza viruses from man.

When did influenza viruses first appear in man? Again,
we haven't a clue. Influenza doesn't remain in a community, but disappears, circulates elsewhere, and then reappears when conditions are favorable. Like the influenza viruses of birds, pigs, and horses, many susceptible humans
are necessary in order to keep the virus active. If we assume that the present behavior patterns of the virus in man
have not changed, then influenza is a relatively recent
event. The old verse about the antiquity of microbes—
"Adam/Had 'em"—probably didn't include the flu viruses. Like smallpox, measles, and other epidemic diseases, influenza activity was unlikely to succeed until the
first large villages were formed about six thousand years

ago. Well-developed trade was also needed to maintain the virus. The influenza virus probably evolved into its present form in man in the past thousand years or so.

Influenza viruses survive by avoiding the antibodies of the creatures they assault. Each time an influenza virus circles the globe, 10 to 30 percent of the human population becomes infected and mounts an antibody defense. A year or so later, when the virus makes another trip around the globe, it finds it harder to replicate and survive, since many people have antibodies and are now immune or resistant to infection. Of course, the flu virus could concentrate on those it missed last time and children born since then. Other viruses do. Measles virus, for example, maintained itself very nicely before vaccine was developed by infecting each new crop of preschoolers.

But the influenza virus prefers a grander style. After a few strenuous trips that meet with antibody resistance, the virus reappears with changes in its surface spikes that the antibodies recognize only vaguely or not at all. The virus is now free to infect the same people again, and so continue on its merry way.

One of the most fascinating characteristics of the influenza A virus is its ability to mutate. Mutations are minor chemical changes occurring naturally during virus reproduction. Picturesquely referred to as genetic "wobble," these mutations account for the fact that of the billions of viruses produced from a single infection, thousands may differ from the others in some subtle characteristics. If the change is too drastic, the virus will not survive. A virus particle unable to attach to a cell because of a mutation in the spikes is, for example, a goner.

Some mutations may be to the advantage of the virus. Influenza A viruses isolated from man do not cause disease in laboratory mice, but they will replicate. Inoculating mice with A virus and allowing the virus to be passed to other mice enables the virus to finally cause a deadly

pneumonia in mice. By this process, scientists are selecting slightly changed viruses that can thrive under the conditions found in the mouse lung. Similar mutations in the
antigens of the surface spikes have a major role in real life.
This is the way the virus overcomes the immunity granted
by previous infections and current vaccinations. The virus
is a master of disguise. Imagine the most wanted criminal,
whose face is on every FBI poster, being able to change his
or her appearance and fingerprints every time the FBI begins to close in. The virus has two mechanisms at its dis-
posal for escaping recognition by the antibody police:
gradual changes (*antigenic drift*) or abrupt changes (*antigenic shift*) in one or both of the two types of surface
spikes.

An antibody that makes a person immune after being
sick with the flu is probably directed against small areas
on the tips of the spikes. Since antibody to the hemagglutinin is principally involved in immunity, small chemical
changes in a few areas on one class of spikes cancel protection. Changes in one or more amino acids, the smallest
building blocks of proteins, probably occur in hundreds of
virus particles among the billions or so produced from
each infection. If there is no immunity to the parent virus,
these few mutants offer no survival advantage and tend to
get lost among their more straitlaced and look-alike broth-
ers and sisters. However, if the infected person has partial
immunity to the parent virus, any virus mutant that differs
in a few amino acids in the crucial hemagglutinin areas
but is normal in all other respects now has the survival advantage. It can multiply and become the predominant virus.

Such gradual antigenic drift can be shown in the laboratory by infecting cells and allowing the "newborn" virus
to emerge into a hostile environment where antibodies
wait. Most of the virus particles will be killed as they
emerge from the cell. But those virus particles that, as a

result of mutation, are even slightly different from their parents survive, reinfect neighboring cells, and thereby prevail. It has not been proven that what occurs in the world is like what we observe in the laboratory, but it seems reasonable. If this process can be demonstrated with a few thousand cells in the laboratory, imagine the opportunity for antigenic drift as the virus infects millions of people throughout the world. With modern techniques scientists can determine which amino acids change and where they are located on the virus spikes. But even armed with this information we do not know how to predict these changes or prevent the consequences.

The higher forms of life have the advantage of sexual reproduction. It is a powerful force in evolution and in survival. An offspring with genes donated by more than one parent has a greater chance of survival. There is a long history of selective breeding dedicated to the development of better crops, hardier livestock, faster horses, and fancier pets. The influenza virus may also have a kind of sexual life.

Recall the description of the eight separate genomes of the influenza virus, each coding for a specific structure or a specific material necessary for replication. If two influenza A viruses enter a cell simultaneously and each starts the replication process, the cell will begin replicating the products specified by the sixteen genomes and also duplicate the genomes themselves. When the offspring from a combination of the two viruses spring from the cell, in theory they may contain the hemagglutinin of one parent and the neuraminidase of the other, and so on for 254 possible combinations. For what we have loosely described here as sex, the scientific term is "genetic reassortment." The effect is an abrupt change in the antigens, or antigenic shift.

Like antigenic drift, antigenic shift is demonstrated in the laboratory. Scientists take advantage of genetic reassortment to breed new influenza viruses with desired features, just as farmers have done with their crops for centuries. Since 1968 all influenza A components of vaccines have been hybrids. They have the desired spikes from the current strains and the high replicative potential from an established laboratory strain. In this way the laborious process of "adapting" a new strain for vaccine production is avoided. This process is unnatural in the sense that scientists are the matchmakers, and the viruses are introduced in a test tube in the vicinity of the cell to be infected.

Genetic reassortment in animals can be shown under more natural experimental conditions. In one elegant test under strict containment conditions, pigs were infected with a human influenza virus (the A/Hong Kong strain); others were infected with the classical swine influenza strain. Both groups were then placed in the presence of uninfected pigs. Within a few days, the innocent bystanders had flu. From many of these pigs, hybrid viruses were obtained that had features of both the human and pig strains.

How often genetic reassortment occurs in nature is not known. We know that human influenza A strains are often recovered from pigs, and that the classical influenza virus of pigs causes disease in man, as seen in the Fort Dix swine flu incident of 1976. In February and March, 1976, the infections at Fort Dix involved both the swine influenza virus and the then-current human A/Victoria virus. All the conditions were present for the creation of a new strain that would have the growth potential of the human strain and the spikes of the swine strain—all the ingredients for a major epidemic. But it didn't happen.

However, in 1977, when mixed epidemics of the Russian flu strains and Victoria flu were prevalent throughout the world, there were several instances when hybrid viruses were recovered. This suggests that at least genetic reassortment among human strains can occur in nature.

Many scientists feel strongly that genetic reassortment is the explanation for the antigenic shift in the Asian virus of 1957 and the Hong Kong virus of 1968. In 1957 both types of spikes changed abruptly. In 1968 only the hemagglutinin changed; the neuraminidase remained the same as in 1976. The possible animal and virus origin of the 1957 strain is a mystery, since no influenza viruses possessing identical antigens have been recovered from animals.

Evidence tracing the cause of the Hong Kong virus is stronger. Similar hemagglutinin antigens were spotted among viruses taken from ducks and horses as early as 1963. This does not mean that either of these species was the donor in 1968, but rather that the virus antigens found in all three species may have come from an unknown common ancestor.

Since 1933, we have witnessed antigenic shifts, in 1957 and in 1968. If genetic reassortment can occur in nature as easily as it does in the laboratory, why are antigenic shifts so infrequent? We don't know how often influenza virus genetic reassortment occurs in nature. Among certain waterfowl it may be a common event and the explanation for the many different subtypes of influenza A viruses found among those species. But in man and other animals it may be an exceedingly rare event.

As long as survival is not threatened by environmental influences, the viruses have no real need for competition from a niece or nephew arising through biparental inheritance. Each virus can do as well as the parent. Therefore, any newcomer that is a little different may be crowded out by the large number of exact copies of the parent. Not so in hard times. As the environmental forces of evil gather in the form of increasing levels of antibodies in the human population, the chances of survival decrease for the current virus and increase for the new kid on the block who has an outside coat that an antibody fails to recognize. This ability to mutate thus makes the influenza virus a formidable foe.

CHAPTER 3

The Flu Virus Gets Around

Watch someone sneeze in bright sunlight and observe the mini-cloud created. We see many droplets, but there are many more we cannot see. With an apparent life of its own, the cloud moves around. The larger particles settle out within a few minutes, but the smaller ones often remain suspended and circulate in the air for hours. If the sneezer is infected with an influenza virus, each droplet could contain hundreds or thousands of virus particles. The next susceptible person stepping into the room enters a cloud of viruses, breathes, and infection is likely to result. Coughing, nose blowing, kissing, and handling contaminated articles can also spread the misery to neighbors.

The influenza virus does not spread as rapidly among family members as we might expect, although families with young children seem to suffer more often from influenza than those without a direct pipeline to school epidemics. We are more likely to become infected at a school, college, prison, hospital, office, or any other closed, poorly ventilated space where people congregate. Shipboard spread of influenza is notorious.

Crowded public transportation has a reputation for spreading disease. The airplane was once suspected of being the ideal environment for spreading influenza. After all, there are hundreds of tired travelers from around the world crowded together in a small space, their mucous membranes irritated by the thin, dry air. But the air exchange in an airplane controls the migration of the viruses. The only recorded incident associating an influenza outbreak with airplane travel occurred in 1976 in Alaska. Because of engine failure, a plane remained on the ground, with crew and passengers aboard, for about four hours. It was cold outside and the doors were kept closed, so the cabin was stuffy. Two days later, after the passengers had reached their destinations, thirty-five of the forty-nine on the flight came down with classic flu. Most of the patients were diagnosed in the laboratory as having had influenza type A. The source of the virus was traced to a young woman who came on board feeling well, but who later developed a cough and fever. Her friends who came to see her off also had influenza the next day.

Endemic influenza describes the occurrence of cases popping up here and there at any time of the year, without any obvious connection among them. Such cases occur through slow, smoldering spread or through reintroduction of viruses from areas of the world where flu is widespread; for example, South America, where winter coincides with our summer.

Epidemic influenza refers to a sharp increase in the number of cases in a given location or region. Usually the influenza virus is similar or closely related to one previously detected in that region.

In a strict epidemiologic sense, a *pandemic* is defined as a series of epidemics that spread rapidly throughout a region or large area(s) of the world. Using that definition, we can say that a pandemic occurs frequently, since it is not unusual for an influenza virus to circle the globe, causing disease, in a period of less than a year. Therefore, the term "pandemic influenza" is reserved to describe the rapid

global spread of the disease caused by influenza A virus
originating through an antigenic shift—that is, through a
complete and abrupt change in one or both types of its surface spikes. Before the days when the virus could be isolated and studied in the laboratory, epidemiologists included in their definition of the pandemic effects upon
general mortality rates. Since influenza B viruses are not
known to undergo antigenic shifts, they cause only endemic or epidemic influenza.

Endemic influenza is virtually impossible to detect
without laboratory assistance. Since so many agents cause
respiratory disease, an occasional uncomplicated influenza may resemble illnesses caused by many of these
agents, and vice versa. Even in years when there is no laboratory evidence of an influenza virus epidemic, the National Center for Health Statistics reports cases of influenza. Who is right—those who consider influenza a
clinical term to describe a disease caused by many agents
or those who consider influenza a term to be used only to
describe those illnesses known to be caused by influenza
A and B viruses? We prefer the latter, since it makes the
problem scientifically clearer. But it doesn't help the physician who hasn't the time, resources, or inclination to request laboratory confirmation of every case diagnosed
clinically as influenza.

If we consider the total number of all viral-like respiratory diseases on an annual basis, influenza viruses may account for no more than 10 percent for adults and less than
that for children. If, however, we limit the cases to respiratory illnesses that can, in two to three weeks, disable entire
sports teams, three-quarters of the cadets at West Point,
one-half of the students of a school, and one-quarter of
your friends, only influenza will be on the list. This characteristic makes influenza A and B viruses different from
all other respiratory disease agents, giving us a basis for
monitoring influenza.

Sharp increases in absenteeism from work or school, increased visits to doctors' offices and clinics, and increased hospitalization often are signs of influenza, but not always. During some years school and industrial absenteeism did not increase dramatically in spite of laboratory evidence of the presence of influenza A and in spite of a sharp increase in visits to medical facilities. In other years, outbreaks occurred in some schools and other institutions, but not in those being monitored.

Since there is no legal requirement to report influenza cases, the Public Health Service (PHS) relies heavily on information obtained through the cooperation of state health departments. When possible, the states provide data on pneumonia and influenza admissions, emergency room visits to key hospitals in large cities, and school and industrial absenteeism. The information, however, varies in quality from state to state and provides only a rough estimate of sickness in the United States. Most states also support a laboratory surveillance program in cooperation with the WHO Influenza Center at the Center for Disease Control (CDC). These laboratories report the number of specimens received from cases of respiratory disease as well as the number of viruses isolated and the serologic diagnoses made each week. These laboratory data confirm the identity of the reported outbreaks and provide information on the extent and duration of the epidemic. More specific information on infection rates, the age of those attacked, and the impact of the virus on the community requires special studies.

To provide a more consistent index of influenza activity, the Public Health Service depends on the concept of excess mortality. Simply put, the number of pneumonia/influenza deaths will inflate the number of total deaths above the number expected during a nonepidemic period. No other event except a heat wave can have this effect. From this simple basis, a rather complicated statistical formula was developed to predict a typical number of week ⌣ deaths, based on the reports from the last five influenza-free years. The Office of Vital Statistics in 121 American cities of over 100,000 people reports to CDC each week the total number of deaths and the deaths where influenza or pneumonia are listed on the certificate as causes. Statistics from about one-third of the nation's population are fed weekly into the computer and compared with normal values. An increased number of deaths over at least a two-week period strongly indicates an influenza epidemic in that region. The excess mortality measurement is two to four weeks behind the clinical and documented laboratory evidence of influenza A and sometimes influenza B. This lag period is always present and is probably caused by the duration of illness before death or by the time required for the flu to spread from the younger, more mobile generation to the elderly and infirm.

The excess mortality figures and the number of deaths attributed to influenza are only estimates. Too often we fall into the trap of taking excess death figures literally, perhaps because they're the only data we have. The numbers are reasonable estimates, but we still can't state for certain, as the newspapers do, that 24,800 persons died of influenza in 1973.

The accuracy of excess death figures has been questioned by some epidemiologists for three reasons. First, preliminary numbers published by the CDC are projected from only one-third of the nation to the entire nation; large errors are therefore possible. Second, reports from the 121 cities reflect urban, not rural, deaths; therefore, estimates can be higher than actual. Third, the norm, or expected number, of pneumonia deaths is based on figures from a few years back, when pneumonia was more frequent; therefore, the actual number of excess pneumonia deaths could be higher than estimated.

Except for certain facts, such as age and sex, we know

e people who make up the excess death sta-
vhat caused their deaths. It is assumed that
total excess deaths, usually three times that
a and influenza deaths, represent deaths
mainly from cardiovascular disease complicated by influenza, but we can't be certain. Clearly, excess deaths during an influenza epidemic is a validated phenomenon. We
need only to remember that the purpose of the excess
death figures is to document the impact of the epidemic,
not to provide a precise body count. Final excess death figures are calculated about three years after an epidemic
from data supplied by the National Center for Health Statistics from a scientifically designed 10 percent sample
representing a cross section of the nation. We think this
method is more accurate, but it's still an estimate.

The most severe pandemic in modern times occurred in
1957–58. The virus, now called the Asian (H2N2) strain,
possessed spikes that were totally different from those
found in previous influenza A strains. We aren't certain of
the origin of the virus, but it was first recognized in central
China in February 1957. It spread rapidly to Hong Kong,
Malaysia, Taiwan, and other neighboring countries. During late May, it was recovered from travelers returning to
the United States. At nearly the same time, outbreaks were
reported from countries in Europe and the Middle East.
Extensive epidemics occurred in the Southern Hemisphere in July and August. Epidemics in the Northern
Hemisphere began to spread in late September, with peak
activity in October. The virus caused epidemics in nearly
every major country in the world within six months after it
reached Hong Kong. By early 1958, second waves of influenza were reported by many countries in the Northern
Hemisphere. During the first and second waves in the
United States, perhaps as many as 60 million people were
affected with an estimated excess mortality of nearly
70,000.

In 1968–69 the virus referred to as the Hong Kong (H3N2) flu appeared. It possessed only one new surface antigen, unlike its predecessors. Like the 1957 strain, it emerged in the Far East, but unlike 1957, it was seen in China in July about the same time it was reported in Hong Kong. Its true geographic origin is anyone's guess. Like the 1957 strain, it spread rapidly around the world. Unlike the 1957 strain, it caused major epidemics that year only in certain areas. The United States was one of the first countries in the Northern Hemisphere to report a nationwide epidemic, which began in October. By the end of 1968, the virus had struck an estimated 30 million persons in the United States, and the excess mortality was figured at slightly over 30,000. Epidemics were still being reported in the Southern Hemisphere in mid-1969 and in Europe during the fall and early winter of the same year, more than a year after the virus was detected in Hong Kong.

Why the Hong Kong virus did not behave like the 1957 pandemic virus is not known. The most frequent explanation for the less-than-ferocious nature of the Hong Kong virus is that only one surface antigen was new, the hemagglutinin. The other type of spike, the neuraminidase, remained substantially unchanged for ten years. Although antibody against the neuraminidase provides less protection than antibody against the hemagglutinin, nearly everybody had neuraminidase antibody, and perhaps that was enough to slow the spread of the virus as well as to lessen the severity of the disease.

The reduction of excess mortality, but not of virus spread, could have been due to the fact that people born before the turn of the century had antibody to the Hong Kong virus. Therefore, unlike the 1957 pandemic when the excess mortality increased with increasing age, the excess mortality in 1968–69 leveled off at age sixty-five and decreased in individuals of increasing age. Antibody resulting from a virus infection over a half-century earlier still provided some protection. Another thought bearing on the lower virulence of the Hong Kong virus suggests that the severe H2N2 epidemics experienced worldwide in the winter/spring of 1967–68 dampened the spread of the new pandemic strain in 1968–69.

If we stick with our definition of a pandemic, we can identify only two (1957 and 1968) since the first isolation of the virus from man in 1933. Even then, to accept the 1968 outbreak as a pandemic requires a stretch of the imagination.

Most textbooks assert that an influenza pandemic occurs every ten to eleven years. The test of the truth of that statement is limited by our knowledge of the virus, which extends over a period of only forty-five years. We can date the beginning of our awareness a little further back by using the technique of seroarchaeology. That word will not be found in any dictionary. It is laboratory jargon for reaching into the past by examining the sera from older persons for evidence of previous influenza infections. The technique assumes that people retain high levels of antibody throughout life, and often the highest levels against the influenza virus that caused their very first infection, usually by age three. By testing the sera from persons of different ages against various influenza viruses, antibody patterns can be detected that identify periods of virus dominance. Using this technique, we can show that the virus of the 1918 pandemic was closely related to the virus that was first isolated from pigs in 1930. Whether or not the viruses were identical is not relevant. The fact is that a virus closely related to the swine virus first appeared in the human population in 1918.

We can also show that a virus with hemagglutinins closely related to those of the Hong Kong virus was present about the turn of the century. We can't be certain, but it is likely that the first introduction of this virus into the human population resulted in the pandemic of 1891–92.

Thus, from 1890 to 1976 we have strong evidence of antigenic shifts in the hemagglutinin in 1889, 1918, 1957, and 1968. These findings coincide with the three most severe epidemics thought to be caused by influenza over the last one hundred years—those of 1889–92, 1918–19, and 1957–58.

The immunologic and genetic evidence shows that the influenza A viruses from 1918 through 1956 all belong to the same family, not three (Hsw1N1, HON1, and H1N1), as originally proposed. We can't be certain about the viruses from 1889 to 1918. But from even the limited data since 1918 we must conclude that antigenic shifts and pandemics have not occurred every ten to eleven years as is commonly quoted, but rather at intervals of thirty-nine and eleven years.

Substantial support for the swine flu program in 1976 came from those who felt that the Fort Dix outbreak of swine influenza signaled the rebirth of the dangerous 1918 virus—right on schedule. The virus didn't appear. Obviously there are flaws in the recycling theory. Evidence of previous circulation of the Asian strain is based on the finding of low levels of antibody in considerably less than half of those in the proper age group. But if such a virus was in circulation, it was only remotely related to the Asian strain. Although the serologic evidence for previous circulation of the Hong Kong (H3) antigen is overwhelming, it could not have been the same virus as in 1968, since additional serologic evidence indicates that the neuraminidase of the first virus was similar to that of a virus from horses, and not similar to that of the Hong Kong virus. Influenza viruses with antigens similar to those previously seen can recur, but there is no evidence that these events have any predictable sequence or periodicity.

Having written all of this, we will add further to the complexity by pointing out that the "Russian" flu virus which appeared in 1977 represents an antigenic shift. The

surface antigens (H1N1) are different from the previously
prevalent Victoria or Texas H3N2 strains. This current
H1N1 strain was first identified in northeast China in May
1977. It spread southward through the remainder of China
from July to November. In November the virus caused outbreaks in the Soviet Union and Hong Kong. By mid-
December it covered the Soviet Union, and by mid-
January it had reached eastern Europe, England, and
Singapore. The first recognized outbreak in the United
States occurred in a high school in Cheyenne, Wyoming,
in mid-January. One month later, outbreaks of the virus
struck almost every military base in the country. Attack
rates as high as 73 percent were reported by many institutions. By the end of March, nearly every state suffered outbreaks of the virus.

Although the virus represented an antigenic shift, it
could hardly be labeled a pandemic strain. There were no
increases in industrial absenteeism, no whole families
stricken, no increased hospitalizations, and no excess
mortality. Because the virus was nearly identical to the
one that circulated in the early 1950s, practically no one
over the age of twenty-five was infected in 1978. Further-
more, the Russian H1N1 strains have not replaced the
Hong Kong H3N2 strains. As late as 1981–82 both subtypes were in circulation throughout the world. This is an
unprecedented event in the chronicle of influenza.

Considerable controversy exists over the origin of the
H1N1 strain. Some propose that the strain originated by
accident from a laboratory freezer, because of the unlikeli-
hood that this virus could reside in nature for more than
twenty-five years and appear with essentially the same genetic characteristics. We do not know the origin of the virus. There may be a mechanism for dormancy that we do
not understand. We cannot be certain of the basis for any
antigenic shift. Only time will tell whether the H1N1 virus
fits anybody's theories of influenza virus periodicity, re-

cycling, or pandemics, or whether we will have to generate a new set of theories.

The pattern seems logical. The pandemic virus emerges, propagates rapidly throughout the world, completely crowds out the previously prevalent virus, and causes widespread epidemics and sharp increases in excess deaths. Afterwards, the same virus, and later its progeny, return periodically and cause epidemics, until they are replaced by the next pandemic strain. At least this is the apparent epidemiologic pattern for the years 1918–1956, and certainly for the years 1957–67 and from 1968 to the present.

Epidemics of influenza A virus flourished in the United States in seven of the last ten years. Epidemics of influenza B virus are seen frequently but are not widespread and affect mostly children. Influenza B epidemics may sometimes produce excess mortality rates, but not very high nor often. Appendix 1 lists the epidemics of influenza A and B viruses recorded in the United States during the years from 1957 to 1976.

Rarely a year goes by without some influenza activity in the United States. Epidemics and their accompanying excess deaths have occurred fourteen times in the last twenty years. Scientists say these frequent epidemics result from gaps in immunity and drifts in the antigenic composition of the virus. That sounds logical, but let's examine how much blame can be placed on us and how much on the virus. And we want to add a third factor to the equation—virus virulence.

Most immunity is found in those who previously were infected with the currently prevalent virus. Considering the statistics on attack rates and school absenteeism and the reports in the newspapers headlined "Flu Hits City," it may be difficult to imagine how there could be many gaps in immunity following a pandemic. The dramatic outbreaks, not the final assessments, grab the headlines and mold many opinions. In 1968–69 the Hong Kong virus neither caused 50 percent absenteeism in every school nor affected every community equally. A "hit and miss" epidemic is more characteristic of influenza. For the entire country, the estimated clinical attack rate, that is, people who were actually ill, was 15 percent. If we assume that the infection rate (people who were infected but may or may not have been ill) was, as is typical, nearly double the clinical rate, then a maximum of 30 percent of the population was infected with the Hong Kong virus during that first year. More than two-thirds were still susceptible. Millions of new susceptibles are added through births to the population each year. Through waning immunity, unknown millions in the "immune" group may become susceptible to reinfection (but not necessarily illness) each year, and since infection rates during subsequent epidemics have been on the order of 15 to 20 percent, then three to four more epidemics with the Hong Kong virus might easily occur.

The importance of antigenic drift for virus survival during the early interpandemic years is not clear. The Asian virus, after its debut in 1957, returned with little or no evidence of antigenic drift and caused epidemics of varying severity in 1959, 1960, and 1962. On the other hand, the Hong Kong virus, after its introduction in 1968–69, returned only in 1970, with no evidence of antigenic drift. Thereafter, Hong Kong viruses of moderate drift caused the epidemic in 1972–73 (the England strain), and viruses exhibiting still greater drift were responsible for the epidemics of 1973–74 (the Port Chalmers strain), 1975–76 (the A/Victoria strain), and 1977–78 (predominantly the A/Texas strain).

The epidemic influenza A (H1N1) virus of 1956–57 bears little resemblance to its probable parent of nearly forty years earlier. The H2N2 virus of 1967–68 appears to be only distantly related to its parent of 1957. Perhaps drift may achieve the same result as shift. Probably not, even though the virus survives well enough. The drift is gradual and is therefore reflected in the antibody patterns of the population following each epidemic. The evolving virus is never totally new.

Virus virulence is another factor to include in the epidemic equation. We know that naturally occurring avian influenza viruses with identical antigens can vary widely in their ability to sicken and kill chickens or turkeys. We know that the current H1N1 virus, unlike the H3N2 viruses, causes little or no serious disease in the age group most susceptible, those under twenty-five. In many respects, influenza B seems less virulent than influenza A. One explanation for the 1918 debacle suggests that the virus was of unusual virulence. Everyone agrees that a minimum level of virulence is essential if the virus is to survive; whether the virus in humans sometimes exceeds that minimum is difficult to prove. Humans and chickens don't react in the same ways. It is impossible to study separately each factor that contributes to an epidemic. From animal studies we know that virulence and antigens are not linked, but even the most virulent virus for humans can't achieve its deadly potential if most of the population has some immunity to it. Immunity is variable; antigens drift, and virulence is complicated. Conditions required for an epidemic are complex. The virus, the host, and perhaps even environmental forces not yet considered (such as severe weather, air pollution, crowding, and population movement) may be factors.

It is startling to note that the number of excess deaths estimated between the pandemic years exceeds that estimated for the pandemic years. For example, excess deaths estimated for 1957–58 were nearly 70,000. The ten-year interpandemic period that followed recorded 144,000 excess deaths. Similarly, the 1968 pandemic caused an estimated 33,000 excess deaths, but interpandemic viruses up to the present time caused more than three times that number. Sickness rates from influenza during the interpandemic years are often very high. The pandemic represents only the beginning.

One final note—the death rate from influenza and pneumonia has steadily declined since the 1930s. Reasons are complicated and include the use of antibiotics to control secondary bacterial infections, better general health, and improved medical care of the elderly. It is hoped that this trend will continue and that influenza will become a less serious public health problem. We can't be sure. Human and domestic animal populations are increasing, human population centers have shifted, and modern transportation has increased the possibility for global virus spread. Recall that from 1840 through the 1880s, influenza disappeared as a recognizable epidemic disease, only to reappear and cause a major pandemic in 1889–90.

CHAPTER 4

Keeping Track of a Formidable Foe

Isolationism has been a tempting political philosophy during many periods of our history. Even today, when the going gets tough, there are strong sentiments for us to withdraw and let the rest of the world solve its problems. But again and again our nation learns the value of being open to interacting with other countries on issues of common interest.

The elimination of yellow fever from the urban centers of the tropical and semitropical areas of the world is a superb example of the value of international cooperation. As a result of the same cooperation, travelers to most parts of the world no longer fear major epidemic disease. Ending the scourge of smallpox could not have been achieved without coordinating the public health talents and resources of both developed and developing countries. This feat was accomplished during the period 1967–78 by the World Health Organization, through the cooperation of countries that were, in other ways, at odds. There were many wars going on, both hot and cold, but in the eradication of smallpox, each country fought a common enemy.

Following the wily influenza virus requires a highly sophisticated network of international cooperation. No one escapes influenza, and the formation of an influenza surveillance program was one of the first acts of the World Health Organization when it was established in 1947. After a modest beginning, over seventy countries now participate in the program.

The network gives an early warning of new or altered influenza virus subtypes, wherever they occur. In this way vaccines can be produced with minimal delay. In effect, scientists keep an international journal of the global where, when, and what of influenza viruses, striving constantly to understand the strange ways of the virus and the origins of pandemic disease.

The World Health Organization in Geneva is the hub of the efforts to keep track of our formidable foe. There are no laboratories there nor are there any influenza laboratories anywhere operated by WHO. Geneva makes things happen by getting nations to work together against a common enemy. Laboratories in London (National Institute for Medical Research) and Atlanta (Center for Disease Control) serve as international centers. Each center deals directly with laboratories around the world whose facilities vary from primitive to highly sophisticated.

Since influenza ranks low among health priorities in the developing countries, and because the vaccines prepared with viruses from these countries benefit only the "rich" countries, some young countries could feel exploited. WHO understands this and encourages participation by providing the supplies for laboratories. In turn, the recipients expedite the forwarding of findings to the appropriate center and to Geneva.

This international venture depends upon dedicated people. Fortunately, in many developing countries there are scientists and physicians who support the principles of public health in spite of poor pay, small budgets, and infinite red tape. It is these people who establish sentinel populations in military barracks, schools, and hospitals, and who sustain personal ties with practicing physicians in order to detect the first hint of influenza.

Let's look at how the virus surveillance works in practice, beginning with the report of influenza in a small country in South America. The first signs of the influenza season may come to the attention of the head of the virology laboratory, whom we shall call Dr. Lopez, via a friend who is a clinic physician. The physician reports that he thinks he saw several cases of influenza among those attending the out-patient clinic that morning. He asks Dr. Lopez for the special fluid for collecting specimens for virus isolation. Dr. Lopez drops by the clinic on his way home that afternoon and leaves several vials of collection fluid and forms for recording patients' histories.

The next morning at the clinic, two more influenzalike respiratory infections are seen. Specimens are collected from the nose and throat of each patient with small, dry cotton swabs attached to applicator sticks. The sticks are broken off, the swabs are dropped into the collection fluid, and the fluid is immediately placed in the refrigerator. At the same time, a blood sample is taken.

The specimens are soon delivered to Dr. Lopez at the virology laboratory. There the virus specimens are quickly treated with a mixture of antibiotics intended to stop the overgrowth of bacteria normally found in the throat. Viruses are not affected by these antibiotics. With the decks cleared, the clotted blood specimens are put in the centrifuge to separate the red blood cells from the straw-colored serum. After ten to fifteen minutes, the technician removes the serum from the packed blood clots, places it in sterile vials labeled with the patients' names, and stores it in a freezer for future use.

In the meantime, Dr. Lopez collects several chicken eggs from his incubator. Each egg contains a living embryo ten to twelve days old. (Chicks hatch at twenty-one days.) Dr. Lopez also visits another incubator to obtain tissue cultures of human cancer cells. In this case, the cells came from a human skin cancer and have been grown in the laboratory for years. He injects small amounts of the virus specimen into several chick embryos, covers the needle hole in the eggshell with glue or wax to prevent bacterial contamination, and places the egg in an incubator set at a temperature similar to that of the nasal passages, about four degrees lower than normal body temperature. If the virus is there, it will be warm and happy and will surely multiply in the cells covering the embryo. With a pipette, he places fluid from the same virus specimens in a test tube with cancer cells and puts the test tubes in the same incubator.

Daily, Dr. Lopez or his technician observes the cell cultures through a microscope, looking for any unusual changes in the appearance of the cells. Two days after inoculation, he removes the eggs from the incubator and places them in the refrigerator overnight to kill the embryo and prevent bleeding when the eggs are broken open and the fluids collected. The next day a drop of fluid from each egg and an equal amount of chicken or human red blood cells are placed in test tubes. After an hour, Dr. Lopez holds up the tubes to the light and in this case he decides that no virus is present or that, if it is, its concentration is too low to be detected by the clumping of red blood cells. He then reinoculates to try again.

By the end of the week, the eggs have not revealed the presence of an influenza virus; however, the cancer cell cultures are beginning to show destructive changes typical of some viruses. Dr. Lopez immediately repeats the test to confirm these observations.

Ten days after the collection of the first specimens, Dr. Lopez drops by the clinic to tell his physician friend that flu virus was not recovered from either patient, but that another virus was isolated from one of them. From his experience in "reading" virus-infected cells, Dr. Lopez is certain that the virus is an adenovirus, a common cause of respiratory disease. He can't be sure which of the many types of adenovirus it is until further tests, requiring weeks, are done. Since adenoviruses may be carried in the tonsils for years after the initial infection, Dr. Lopez can't be sure that this is the virus that caused this person's illness until after he tests the patient's convalescent serum for antibodies.

The physician arranges to have a blood sample collected from each of the patients three weeks after they first experienced symptoms of illness. By this time, one patient has been completely recovered for two weeks, but the young man from whom the adenovirus was isolated is still feeling tired and has a slight cough. In the laboratory the serum is separated as before.

The first serum specimen, called *acute* since it was taken at the first sign of illness, and the second serum specimen (*convalescent*) from each patient are tested for antibodies against many infectious marauders that can cause respiratory disease. This is an important test, since by this time acute and convalescent serum pairs from other clinics and hospitals have also been submitted for testing. A diagnosis requires demonstration of an increase in antibodies (between acute and convalescent serum pairs) against a suspected infectious agent. From the test results the next day, Dr. Lopez sees no increase in adenovirus antibodies in the convalescent serum from the patient from whom the adenovirus was isolated. However, the adenovirus antibodies in the acute and convalescent sera are high. This suggests to Dr. Lopez that the patient had a recent adenovirus infection but that infection was not the cause of his most recent episode of respiratory disease. Analyzing the test further, he sees no changes in antibody to other known infectious agents of the respiratory tract, including the parainfluenza viruses, respiratory syncytial virus, influenza viruses, or psittacosis agent. However, against *Mycoplasma pneumonia* there is 128 times more antibody in the convalescent than in the acute serum. This agent was clearly the cause of the patient's illness. Infection from this invader accounts for the prolonged recovery period and residual hacking cough. The patient probably had a slight pneumonia that was unrecognized because no chest X-rays were taken.

The rest of the serologic tests were routine for this time of the year. Several young patients showed increases in antibody because of parainfluenza type-three virus and respiratory syncytial virus, but most of the sera were negative. No patient showed any evidence of influenza virus infections.

Sometimes Dr. Lopez finds these negative tests discouraging. The patients have a respiratory disease—many of which are influenzalike—yet his laboratory can rarely identify the specific cause in more than one-quarter of the cases. He knows that even the best virus laboratories in the world often don't exceed a diagnostic rate of 50 percent, but he is also concerned that his batting average is low simply because he doesn't have everything needed.

Most of the developed countries use fresh cell cultures prepared from kidneys of rhesus monkeys as their mainstay for isolating viruses. But monkeys are expensive and are rarely available. Previously, many laboratories, including his own, used cell cultures prepared from kidneys of spontaneously aborted human fetuses or from babies that had died at birth. Public attitudes toward the use of human tissue for scientific purposes has changed over the years, and now legal requirements and red tape make the use of human tissue virtually impossible.

Without fresh primate cells, the laboratory must rely on more easily obtainable cell cultures, mostly of cancer cells. In spite of their ominous character, they are easy to grow and maintain in the laboratory. Unlike fresh primate cells, cancer cells will grow forever, but will not isolate as many viruses as fresh primate cell cultures. Tests for serum antibody are also dependent upon the number of viruses that can be grown by the lab. Therefore, the laboratory is frustrated in the service it can provide. Fortunately, these cells will isolate polio viruses, and that is one service that Dr. Lopez is confident they provide well.

Dr. Lopez's depression does not linger. Two weeks later he learns from the hospital at a nearby army recruit training base that admissions for an influenzalike disease have doubled during the last three days. He is confident that this disease is influenza. And it is. Dr. Lopez and his technicians inject twelve eggs with nose and throat samples collected from patients at the recruit training base. Within three days, they isolate five viruses identified as influenza type A viruses. That same day, after further testing, Dr. Lopez notifies the army hospital by phone that the outbreak was caused by an influenza A virus similar to strains prevalent last year. He reports his findings to the Ministry of Health and speculates that, because the virus looks like last year's, no major epidemics should be anticipated, but that local outbreaks and epidemics are possible.

Dr. Lopez reports his findings to the WHO Influenza Center in Atlanta and the WHO headquarters in Geneva. Because the viruses do not appear to be appreciably different, he economizes by using air mail instead of a telegram. He inoculates eggs with the viruses several more times to increase their concentration and capacity to replicate. Two weeks after the viruses are first isolated, he sends a sample by air mail to the Atlanta laboratory for further study.

Each virus isolated in the laboratory, no matter what the source, is called a *strain*. Each strain is given a name that lists its type (A, B, or C), where the specimen originated, the laboratory number, the year of isolation, and the subtype of its surface antigens. For example, the fifth influenza A virus, isolated from a clinic in Singapore in 1973, is designated as A/Singapore/5/73(H3N2). Confusing? On the contrary, it is very helpful, and no different from naming children or registering pets. It is a recognition that influenza viruses tend to have distinct personalities and characteristics.

Dr. Lopez's viruses join nearly one thousand strains of viruses already submitted to the center this year from collaborating laboratories throughout the Americas and the Pacific regions. After the viruses are examined in the Atlanta laboratory by the use of more discriminatory reagents, Dr. Lopez's identifications are confirmed as correct. He and the World Health Organization (WHO) in Geneva were told that the strains are similar to those that circulated throughout the world last year.

Most of the strains sent to the Atlanta and London centers are similar this particular year, but not all. About a half-dozen on first screening seem to be different from the others. Even more discriminating tests are needed; therefore, each of these strains is forced into the noses of ferrets. Each virus strain causes disease in the ferrets—fever, sneezing, ruffled fur, and that "worn out" feeling. Two weeks later the technicians collect blood from the recovered animals.

These viruses and their antisera and "reference" viruses and their antisera are compared. Such tests routinely require more than four thousand mixtures of antisera and viruses to be processed in a day. The test shows that at least two of the six viruses in question are quite different from last year's strains. To be certain that these results are correct, the entire effort is repeated the next day. The two strains are indeed different.

Early the next morning the director of the Atlanta center calls the London center director to discuss the two strains that show some antigenic drift from previous strains and to inquire whether the London center has received similar strains from its part of the world. They have not. The directors agree that both centers should be on the lookout. That same day, samples of both the ferret sera and the viruses are sent to London in order to confirm the Atlanta results and to enable the London center to recognize similar viruses if received.

But in less than two weeks, in early August, London calls Atlanta to report that a group of strains has been isolated from an outbreak in New Zealand. These strains might be the next wave of virus. This time London sends several of the strains to Atlanta for confirmation of its results. On the day the samples arrive, the Atlanta center receives reports of a suspected influenza epidemic on Guam. Specimens are on the way. Fortunately, the epidemiologist on Guam is an old hand. The throat and nasal specimens, carefully collected and well packed in dry ice, makes the journey in good shape. Within a week, the center in Atlanta determines that the virus causing the epidemic on Guam is similar to the one causing the outbreak in New Zealand. Atlanta calls London and Geneva to report that the virus is spreading.

Formal reports of the outbreaks in New Zealand and Guam appear in the mid-August edition of the *WHO Weekly Epidemiological Record*, a publication that has air mail distribution to health authorities of all nations. In the next edition, the preliminary laboratory results from London and Atlanta are published, and other centers are encouraged to be on the watch for such strains in their areas. Within the next month, reports of epidemics and shipments of viruses are received from Australia, Singapore, and Hong Kong. Although there is general agreement that this virus represents an antigenic drift, not shift, and that there is little likelihood of a pandemic, clearly the virus will have to be considered as a candidate for next year's vaccine. And the surveillance goes on.

CHAPTER 5

What Happens
When You Get
the Flu

No matter how much you have traveled, there are still places you have only read about and sights and sensations that you have only imagined. The study of biology is similar. Even those who have devoted a lifetime to biology continue to discover in it new sights and sounds and experiences. Of course, there is no Biology Section in the Sunday paper and there are no writers paid to promote the excitement of a human heart in action, the pageantry of white blood cells, or the beat of the ciliated epithelial cells. Ciliated epithelial cells? They're cells located between the nose and the lungs, and they are interesting.

When bits of the lining of the trachea of a chicken or mouse, or any animal that breathes, are placed in a sterile, shallow dish with the proper liquid nutrients, the tissue will remain alive for weeks. During that time, with the aid of an ordinary microscope, one can see the mass of tiny hairs covering the tissue undulate like wind-swept wheat in a field or like sea grass that sways with each incoming wave. These tiny hairs, or cilia, continue to sweep, always in the same direction, day and night, at the same beat. The same action exists throughout the respiratory tract, from the nose to the tiny bronchioles at the entrance to the lungs. Every fraction of a second a wave begins in the bronchioles and travels upward to sweep along a blanket of mucus littered with particles of dust, soot, pollen, bacteria, dead cells, and other debris sucked into our bodies as we breathe. The wave action of the ciliated cells helps clean the respiratory tubules and thus protects us from infection.

Looking like fat columns with thick tufts of hair sticking out of the tops, the ciliated cells rise from a foundation of flat cells with mucus-producing cells scattered throughout. Into this moist, warm environment the influenza virus is inhaled. The virus lands on the mucus blanket and eventually reaches a ciliated cell. In theory the virus, using the enzyme neuraminidase, can dissolve and penetrate the mucus to reach the cell. After attachment, it enters the ciliated cell, and virus replication begins. Within three to four hours, offspring emerge to infect still other ciliated cells. The rate of birth of viruses from each cell peaks about twelve hours after invasion, and viruses quickly spread to virtually every part of the respiratory tract, leaving behind shrunken cells riddled with holes and with unmoving cilia. Damaged and dying cells soon slough off, baring patches of red and swollen throat tissue that offers no protection against the elements or invading bacteria. Without the cleaning action of the cilia, cellular debris accumulates and fluid collects in respiratory passages already narrowed by swelling. Lung cells called alveolar cells are infected by the virus and, like the ciliated cells, are killed. Sometimes alveolar infection occurs before many ciliated cells have been infected.

Continued devastation by the virus could be fatal, but fortunately virus production and spread usually peaks in forty-eight to seventy-two hours and then drops as sharply as it began. It is rare to find a large number of viruses in the respiratory tract more than three to four days after a natural infection.

The sometimes slow road to recovery then begins. Denuded membrane patches in the nose, trachea, bronchi, and bronchioles begin to heal. Newly formed ciliated cells sprout from the basement cells to begin the cleanup process and rid the respiratory tract of its accumulated debris. Depending upon the damage, full repair of the system may require anywhere from a few days to a few weeks.

How does all this affect you? If you are one of the lucky ones, hardly at all. During past epidemics, 30 to 50 percent of the people infected were not ill enough to stay home. In the unlucky ones, the death of cells and the toxic impact of the virus can produce many signs and symptoms.

Listed below are the results of the studies of the symptoms of laboratory-proven influenza virus infections in humans.

	Percent with Symptoms	
RESPIRATORY	Adults	Children
Cough	90	86
Runny nose	82	67
Sneezing	67	38
Sore throat	62	62
Stuffy nose	52	54
Hoarseness	37	22
SYSTEMIC		
Headache	72	81
Feverishness	71	93
Tired-out feeling	67	68
Chilliness	64	37
Muscle ache	62	33
Loss of appetite	37	69
OTHER		
Vomiting	7	26
Nausea	4	23
Diarrhea	0	2

If you check the list, you'll probably find that you experience some of those symptoms at least three to four times a year, particularly during the winter. The symptoms are not all caused by influenza viruses. We play host to many uninvited viruses in our respiratory tract. Some, such as the one hundred different types of rhinoviruses, cause only a common cold. There are several types of coronaviruses that cause more severe colds. About ten kinds of adenoviruses are known to cause respiratory disease. Other viruses, such as the parainfluenza viruses and the respiratory syncytial virus, cause major respiratory illnesses during early childhood, and they can return to infect us later in life. To the list we can add the herpes viruses, enteroviruses, and those bacterialike creatures that behave clinically like viruses, such as mycoplasmas, chlamydia, and now the Legionnaires' disease agent. They add up to more than one hundred thirty-five known organisms that may cause viruslike respiratory disease. Again, these are only the known viruses. At least half of all respiratory illnesses in adults and children cannot be blamed on any known infectious agent. Many unknown agents apparently still exist, and it's little wonder the average person has three to five respiratory infections a year.

Unlike measles and its rash, mumps and its swollen glands, and polio and its useless limbs, there is no single set of signs and symptoms that clearly distinguishes influenza from any other respiratory disease. Further compounding the problem, one person's response to the virus is probably unlike another's, and the response to the next infection may not be like the response to the last.

In spite of all this confusion, some physicians do remarkably well in diagnosing "classical flu," a set of signs and symptoms that is characteristic, but not exclusively, of both influenzas A and B. One morning you may arise feeling at peace with the world, only to find yourself the following morning in the doctor's office with a fever, flushed face, slightly red throat, and complaining of a headache, sore eyes, chills, slight hacking cough, muscle aches, and feeling weak and exhausted. One look at you and the experienced clinician thinks "influenza." Chances are, he or she is right. Proving it, of course, requires a laboratory test.

If your case is uncomplicated, as most are, your fever will break, your headache disappear, and your chills stop within two to three days. But your cough will often continue, your nose run, and the tired feeling persist for one to two weeks longer. You probably won't know how sick you were until you feel better. But in any epidemic the number of people with "classical flu" is no more than a small percentage of people infected with the virus.

Very likely, your child brought the virus home from school. You might recall that his or her illness showed itself, if at all, as only a slight cold, a fever for a day or so. Nothing compared to your bout. Maybe children complain less. We used to think that infants and young children had nothing to fear from influenza. We now know that influenza among the young can be severe, causing croup, bronchitis, and pharyngitis. It is not an illness to be taken lightly.

A fever for four days or longer could mean pneumonia, and it could be fatal. Pneumonia occurs in every age group, but fortunately it is rare. It is more likely to strike those forty-five or older and those with some other complicating diseases that affect the heart, the lungs, or the kidneys. Advancing age does not always mean that influenza will hit harder and that pneumonia will result. Many healthy eighty-year-olds can take influenza in stride. In fact, because of repeated experiences with influenza, they are less likely to become infected than younger people. But when it does strike, older persons are at greatest risk from influenza, partly because they are more likely to have unrecognized chronic diseases that result in complications.

Pneumonia is sometimes caused by the influenza virus itself early in the course of the disease, but usually it is not fatal. The most common form of pneumonia results from bacteria and usually occurs after the patient has won the initial bout with the virus. But when bacteria are the cause, they are almost always the common ones found in the throat, on the skin, or in the intestines. They take advantage of the patient's weakened condition and loss of natural defenses to invade and grow in the lungs, an area normally forbidden to them.

Even now, with a choice of antibiotics available, bacterial pneumonia is a serious disease. Of those patients admitted to hospitals, about one-third die. Many patients who contract pneumonia, however, are already in poor health. In one hospital study, 39 percent of the pneumonia admissions had pre-existing heart disease, 28 percent were alcoholics, 20 percent had chronic lung disease, and 15 percent had diabetes. Hardly a healthy group. Leaving aside the occasional case of viral pneumonia, the typical pneumonia patient hospitalized during an influenza epidemic is no different from one admitted at any other time. Only the number of cases varies.

Influenza virus types A and B are sometimes accused of conspiring with other poorly understood medical problems, such as neurologic disorders, myocarditis, and pericarditis, to mount an attack. More puzzling, however, is the connection of the influenza virus with a disease unrecognized before 1963—Reye's syndrome. This is a mean disease that attacks mostly children. A normal, healthy child with a mild case of influenza appears to recover, when the parents note odd behavior, mainly unusual irritability. With no illness present, the behavior is often ignored. Within days, sometimes hours, irritability gives way to delirium, then to a coma with intermittent convulsions. In spite of the best hospital care and most modern treatment, one-quarter of these children die of brain and liver malfunction. The influenza viruses, as well as the chicken pox virus, appear to trigger the disease, even though they do not actively invade either organ. Beginning with the influenza B epidemic of 1973–74 and subsequent A and B epidemics through 1981 over two thousand cases of Reye's syndrome have been reported in the United States. In 1982, evidence suggesting that aspirin may be a cofactor in this disease led the CDC to advise parents to use caution when administering salicylates (aspirin) to treat children with viral illnesses, particularly chicken pox and influenza-like illnesses. The course of this disease is still not understood.

CHAPTER 6

Take the Flu Bug to Bed

There are libraries chock full of books that give advice on diets to make you healthy, diets to make you skinny, and even diets to make you sexy. There are volumes of advice on living, praying, jogging, working, loving—you name it. Following along in this self-help mode, we can't resist the temptation to offer advice on what you should do about the flu.

We don't understand everything about the virus, but we know a great deal about how influenza affects people. By the time most of us suspect we have the flu, the virus has already infected thousands of cells lining our mucous membranes and produced millions of offspring, all capable of infecting more cells. By the time we sense the consequences of that infection, much of the damage has been done. If we had a miracle drug that could stop all further spread of the virus in the body and if it were taken after the first signs of fever, it might decrease the length of the usual course of uncomplicated illness by a few hours to a day. This would be highly desirable in preventing the more rare complicated forms of the disease. But for the most part, all we can hope for is some relief from the headache, the sore throat, and that aching feeling while we replace our respiratory cells and clean up the virus damage.

All of the advice our mothers gave us applies. Go to bed (that is what you will feel like doing). Don't eat heavy meals (you won't want to, anyway). Drink plenty of fruit juices and liquids (because you will need to replace lost body fluids and salts). Remember the chicken soup and pot liquor and how good they felt going down? Don't smoke (you won't feel like it, anyway). Don't get out of bed until you have at least one day without fever. Even then you may not feel like returning to work or school. Stay in bed or just be lazy for a few days. Through many types of sensations your body will tell you to take it easy.

For most of us, the worst flu will last two or three days. With a few more days to recuperate, we are no worse for the experience. We have even gained some antibodies in the process. Nevertheless, flu is not to be taken lightly. It can be serious for some, even the healthy ones among us. There are several danger signals. Sharp chest pains can mean fluid accumulation in the lungs. A fever of four days or longer can mean secondary bacterial infections leading to bronchitis or pneumonia. So can coughing up phlegm. If you detect any of these signals, contact your physician immediately. Even though antibiotics are not effective against viral diseases, they are effective against bacterial infections that often follow. Prompt medical treatment can prevent the more serious consequences of influenza complications.

You might try to avoid the flu by keeping your distance from the sick, staying away from crowds, driving your car to work instead of taking the bus, and walking up the stairs instead of taking the elevator. But, unless you are a recluse, these tactics probably won't work. The virus is spread not only by people who seem sick, but also by those who appear perfectly healthy. In most communities flu vi-

rus is thoroughly seeded before it erupts
able epidemic.

You might wear a gauze face mask.
Asian countries use them during the res
season even though they probably don't
fortunately, there are not many ways to escape the virus.
Antibody surveys show that sooner or later most of us will
become infected, but not necessarily made ill, by a new
subtype. Because of the ability of the virus to spread unrecognized, quarantine or isolation won't work. We can't
stop the virus from reaching our shores, and we can't prevent it from spreading once it arrives.

We can, however, avoid the most serious consequences
of influenza by maintaining good health. As someone
once said, ''The only way to improve the prisons is to get a
better class of prisoners.'' Our country needs more healthy
people in order to minimize the impact of influenza.

Some people say they never have the flu. It may be true.
Others have viral infections, but never become ill. A few
may never, or hardly ever, become infected. Why? No one
knows. Natural resistance is likely to be a factor.

We know about the resistance mechanisms triggered by
the body as a result of infection. Recall that the virus replication reaches its peak on the second or third day following infection and usually decreases rapidly after that. The
acute symptoms of illness also peak on the second or third
day and generally begin to improve then. The decreases in
both virus replication and illness symptoms occur at a
time when the production of a substance called *interferon*
is reaching its peak in the blood and nasal secretions. This
nonspecific nonantibody substance is suspected to play an
important role in recovery from influenza.

Interferon is a small protein produced by cells infected
with certain viruses. When released from infected cells,
interferon enters surrounding noninfected cells and

...ses them to produce another protein substance that interferes with viral replication. The whole process is like a romantic war story. The outpost (the cell) is invaded by attackers (the virus), and while being hopelessly overrun it bravely manages to send a message to the surrounding uninfected cells to mount their defenses. When the virus reaches the surrounding cells, it takes over the cell processes as usual and begins to make building blocks to produce more of itself. But the forewarned cell defenders sabotage its villainous scheme, and no offspring are launched.

About one week after infection, interferon levels decrease rapidly and antibody is detected in the serum and nasal secretions. At this time, any lingering symptoms of illness or virus replication disappear. Antibody production continues to rise, reaching its peak usually during the second week of infection. Antibodies are produced against antigens and possibly against all viral internal antigenic components as well. Present evidence suggests that only antibodies against the virus surface spikes play a role in protection against disease.

Immunity to infection results from a complex process. Everything operating in the recovery from a viral infection is not fully understood. Antibody is a part of the answer. At the same time that antibody is being produced by one type of lymphocyte, other types of lymphocytes are swinging into action. They attack the virus at the infected cell surface and destroy the infected cell. The lymphocytes send out signals to the "scavenger" cells in the blood to "come clean up the mess." Such cells are involved more in recovery than in protection from influenza virus infection. The chief security against influenza is the antivirus antibodies found in the bloodstream and nasal secretions after an infection.

Evidence shows a strong association between the level of antihemagglutinin antibodies in serum and nasal secre-

tions and protection against influenza. The h
els against the virus, the more solid is the prot
is likely that other unknown factors are invol\

Antibodies contained in fluids from the n
necessarily the same as those produced in ...c bloodstream. Most are produced locally as a result of infection.
Antibody acts by attaching to the virus and preventing its
entry into the cells. In theory, then, these local antibodies
are more important than serum antibodies as the first line
of defense, since the virus lands first on the nasal mucosa
or somewhere in the vicinity. This is difficult to prove,
however, since nearly everyone who has nasal antibody
also has serum antibody.

A number of studies have shown that neuraminidase antibody may afford some protection against infection, but
not much. It seems to be more closely associated with decreased severity of illness. This observation is consistent
with what we know about the behavior of neuraminidase
antibody in laboratory tests. Such antibody will not prevent virus infection but will limit the spread of virus to
other cells.

Synthetic or natural substances for the nonspecific prevention of or intervention in all influenza virus infections
have been widely sought. Interferon has often been touted
as the hope of the future. By the use of synthetic substances, we can cause a cell to produce interferon. But
most of these substances have been too dangerous to be
used in humans. Through the use of modern recombinent
DNA technology interferon for human use can be made
cheaply and in large quantities in bacteria. Additional
studies of the effect of interferon against influenza can be
anticipated.

Antibiotics, of course, are highly effective against bacteria, but not viruses. In the United States only one drug is
licensed to be sold for the prevention of influenza. The
drug, 1–adamantanamine hydrochloride (amantadine),

was developed in the early 1960s by E. I. Du Pont de Nemours and sells under the trade name Symmetrel. It is effective against influenza A. It has no significant impact on type B or other respiratory viruses. Amantadine does not "kill" influenza A viruses but prevents their entry into the cell or the site of infection.

Despite its general availability as a prescription drug, it has not been widely used. Many physicians perhaps recall the unfavorable publicity about the drug when it was approved by the Food and Drug Administration (FDA). There was concern about its side effects and its success in preventing influenza A. Many physicians remember that the Public Health Service recommended against the use of the drug as a substitute for the influenza vaccine in 1968, and that the FDA emphasized that the drug was licensed for use only against the Asian strain, not the new A/Hong Kong strain. As a result, the drug was not used for the prevention of influenza during that period.

Meanwhile, amantadine was found to work wonders in controlling the tremors of Parkinson's disease and was widely prescribed for that purpose. As a consequence, more experience with the drug was gained and other data were generated. In 1976, the drug was approved by the FDA for use against all influenza A viruses.

Amantadine is impressive in laboratory demonstrations. In addition, the 1978 field trials with amantadine proved that the drug was more than 50 percent effective in preventing infection by influenza A H1N1 virus. Those findings, plus the long-term experience with the use of the drug for Parkinsonism, prompted a new look at the potential usefulness of the drug for influenza A.

There is still some concern about amantadine's side effects. The manufacturer issues the following warning:

ADVERSE REACTIONS: The most frequently occurring serious adverse reactions are: depression, con-

gestive heart failure, orthostatic hypotensive episodes, psychosis, and urinary retention. Rarely convulsions, leukopenia, and neutropenia have been reported. Other adverse reactions of a less serious nature which have been observed are the following: hal-
lucinations, confusion, anxiety and irritability; ano-
rexia, nausea, and constipation; ataxia and dizziness
(lightheadedness); livedo reticularis and peripheral
edema. Adverse reactions observed less frequently
are the following: vomiting, dry mouth; headache,
dyspnea; fatigue, insomnia, and a sense of weakness.
Infrequently, skin rash, slurred speech, and visual
disturbances have been observed. Rarely eczematoid
dermatitis and oculogyric episodes have been reported.

Many clinical investigators now feel that the incidence
of side effects from the use of amantadine is not as high as
once thought, and that when adverse reactions do occur,
they are readily reversible by withholding the drug.

At a recent conference a panel of physicians, scientists,
and lay persons reviewed the fifteen years of experience
with amantadine and concluded that the drug had a role in
both the prevention and treatment of influenza A. The priorities for groups to receive the drug for prevention were
listed by the panel as follows:

1. Children and adults at high risk of serious illness or
   death because of underlying illnesses.
2. Adults who have not been vaccinated with an appropriate contemporary influenza vaccine and whose activities are essential to community functions (police officers, firefighters, and selected hospital personnel).
3. Individuals in restricted environments, especially
   older people who have not received vaccines.

The panel recommended that the following groups receive the drug for treatment:

1. The groups listed above.
2. Patients for whom the physician makes the diagnosis of life-threatening primary influenzal pneumonia.
3. Individuals whose positions are essential to community activities; those for whom the shortening of a symptomatic illness by twenty-four hours is judged important.

The panel, however, cautioned that before amantadine is prescribed, there must be both epidemiologic and viralogic evidence of influenza A infection in the community or region. Influenza outbreaks occur in communities over intervals of four to six weeks and may be preceded or followed by outbreaks caused by other viral agents.

Confirming the presence of influenza in the community and distinguishing influenza from respiratory diseases caused by other viruses are easier said than done. With wider acceptance in general medical practice, amantadine could be prescribed for more noninfluenza episodes than for influenza. However, misuse of amantadine for viral disease probably would be far less harmful to the individual and the community than misuse of antibiotics for viral disease.

Let us assume for the moment that the drug can be successful in preventing influenza and that it won't be misused. Can this method of control replace vaccine? Antimalaria drugs, for example, have been highly effective and are widely used. Travelers to the malaria zones of tropical Africa, Asia, and South and Central America have little to fear if they remember to take their daily dose of chloroquine. But unlike malaria, influenza is confined to no well-defined endemic areas and has no predictable time of appearance. For these reasons, the use of the drug for control of influenza in the general population poses enormous practical problems. The population must be warned when the influenza virus is detected in the region. Persons wanting to take the drug must obtain it and pay for it, if not out of pocket, then out of taxes. These people must take the drug daily, without fail, for a period of four to six weeks or longer, until the all-clear signal is sounded. If a person stops taking the drug too soon or travels to another area where flu is still present, infection is possible.

Preventive drugs for any infectious disease have two inherent disadvantages: cost and the potential for selecting mutual strains that can overcome the effects of the drug. Reports of chloroquine-resistant strains of the malaria parasites, for example, are increasing at an alarming rate. Consequently, even for malaria, the replacement of preventive drugs with an effective vaccine is a major goal. We have much to learn about drugs, particularly those intended to combat influenza viruses.

CHAPTER 7

The Swine Flu Affair

In mid-January 1976, during the postholiday slump, an influenzalike epidemic abruptly struck army recruits at Fort Dix, New Jersey. That incident marked the beginning of what has been variously described as the swine flu "fiasco," "debacle," "disaster," or, more kindly, "the swine flu affair." It is not our intention to fault or defend the decision to vaccinate nearly 213 million Americans against swine flu. As with most controversial issues, there are good arguments on both sides. A bold, imaginative step to some is a fiasco to others. It will be useful to briefly review the events surrounding this unprecedented program and glean any guidance it offers for the future.

It takes a lab test to be sure about flu. Specimens from the epidemic may not have been analyzed if the state's chief epidemiologist had not bet the senior army doctor that there was flu at Fort Dix. It was just a friendly professional wager about an ordinary medical episode. However, when the New Jersey state laboratory confirmed several cases of flu caused by the dominant Victoria virus, it also discerned other cases of flu which were not caused by that virus. An unidentified virus was isolated from four cases, including a fatality, and sent to CDC for identification. On February 12, in the evening, the CDC determined the unknown agent to be the swine flu virus. This was totally unexpected.

On the basis of serologic tests, it had been known for years that the virus found in swine was closely related to the virus that appeared to have caused the 1918 pandemic. Because the virus had been present for years in pigs, it was assumed that it was no longer a danger to humans. The outbreak at Fort Dix suggested that the virus was again a threat, but the return of swine flu was anything but certain. Laboratory tests cannot determine viral virulence, and so the uncertainty was compounded. It was clear, however, that the issue demanded close attention.

Four swine flu cases did not make an epidemic, so careful surveillance and data-gathering began. A fifth soldier who had been sick in early February was identified as a swine flu victim, and through blood samples eight more cases were identified. Working from the results of antibody tests on recruits, investigators speculated that as many as several hundred more recruits had been infected by the swine flu virus.

By the beginning of March, usually the last month of the flu season, the only signs of the swine flu epidemic in the world were at Fort Dix. But the possibility of a swine flu outbreak in the future could not be disproved. What could not be disproved must be allowed for. Most of the scientists were well aware of the professional risks they incurred if they mounted a national immunization program and the virus did not appear. Most were equally aware of their responsibility for the public's safety in the event of an epidemic. Something had to be done. The only question was how to proceed.

The CDC considered the options: "minimum response," in which the government assisted in financing shots for everyone through normal channels; a "government program," in which federal and state agencies would purchase the vaccine and act without the participation of private physicians; and the program finally recommended by CDC—federal purchase of vaccine for everyone, vaccine production by private manufacturers, and immunization through a mix of public-private services. Included—but discounted—was the "do nothing" option.

This major health issue, requiring spending a lot of money, came up through channels to the Department of Health, Education, and Welfare (HEW). The CDC recommendations were endorsed by the assistant secretary for Health and the secretary of HEW.

The HEW request for extra money to run a swine flu immunization program reached President Gerald Ford on March 15. It was clear that a no-win decision must be made. If there were no pandemic, the inoculated population might be bitterly resentful. And if the pandemic struck, all efforts would not likely be enough. But the CDC and HEW positions removed the choice of doing nothing.

President Ford and most of his advisors viewed the issue as a simplistic, nonpolitical choice but postponed a decision until other experts were consulted on March 24. At that time, Ford listened to opinions on the danger of the disease, the importance of educating the public, the harmlessness of the vaccine, and advantages of closing the "antigenic gap" in our population. In the absence of any advice to the contrary, Ford made the decision—allocate the money and proceed with the vaccination of every man, woman, and child in the United States against swine flu.

With the president's announcement on March 24 that he was asking Congress to appropriate $135 million for the program, dissenters began to surface. Nevertheless, the money for the program was swiftly appropriated by Congress. The hearings that were held seemed only to expedite the process. The goal of inoculating 95 percent of all

Americans was set, although most health professionals thought it unrealistic.

Vaccine production began, and field trials were planned. The trials began on April 21 with the arrival of experimental batches of vaccine prepared in several different ways by manufacturers. The vaccines were tested using one dose per subject. When the results of the field trials were revealed on June 21 and 22, it was clear that for persons under eighteen, the vaccine from two manufacturers caused too many fevers and sore arms. Only the vaccine from two other manufacturers could be used. In addition, for all persons under twenty-four, two doses would be required. More field trials would be needed to find out the results of second doses. The necessity of second doses for young adults and children also raised the probability that the amount of vaccine that would be necessary had been underestimated.

Another debate was going on. Should the vaccine be given in the absence of any further evidence of swine flu in the world or should it be stored in warehouses until further evidence was available? Those who felt it should be stored in warehouses argued that the vaccine would be less effective if given this year and the epidemic appeared next year. In addition, the epidemic may not appear at all. Those who felt the vaccine should be given now argued that the time from detection of another outbreak to a full-blown epidemic would be too short to immunize everyone if the vaccine were stored in a warehouse. They felt the vaccine would be better stored in people, not warehouses. Early immunization won the day, but the media emphasized the controversy, not the agreement.

The list of problems lengthened. Word came that no insurance company wanted to insure the manufacturers of the vaccine, and without that backup, no vaccine would be bottled. The insurance industry insisted that the danger

of extensive liability claims was both enormous and unpredictable.

The delay and ultimate rescue of the swine flu program
is a story within a story. It began in the early 1960s when
large court awards were being given to people suing because of adverse side effects attributed to immunization
shots. In a case against Wyeth, the polio vaccine manufacturer, $200,000 was awarded to an eight-month-old infant
who contracted polio after receiving live-virus vaccine.
The circuit court upheld the award, and the Supreme
Court refused to hear the case even though Wyeth had included a warning in the shipping carton and experts testi-
fied that the case was not vaccine-related.

The vaccine court settlement trend was threatening to
the nervous vaccine manufacturers, and they looked to the
government to both warn the public of any dangers and
deal with any victims of the vaccine. Although everyone
agreed that the vaccine was safe, the insurance manage-
ment took a very different view. With 200 million doses,
there were bound to be many lawsuits. Many of these
would be without foundation, but even with no court
award, the overhead costs looked impossible. No
insurance—not at any price!

In late June, the House Health Subcommittee held hearings on an HEW plan to indemnify the swine flu program.
The Congress was very unsympathetic. On June 19, President Ford was consulted. He asked for another assessment
of the danger and was told that while a pandemic was possible, the probability of it was unknown. There was no
willingness to suggest the probability of danger was past
in spite of the absence of additional cases since January.

President Ford had no choice. He put on the pressure;
all parties maneuvered a bit more; and then a totally unexpected event tipped the balance. In the first week of August "legionnaire's disease" caught national attention.

The fact that the swine flu virus was initially suspected as the culprit probably helped. The legionnaire's disease headlines cut off debate in Congress. On August 12, President Ford signed the bill that made the swine flu program possible.

The government picked up the tab for coverage for swine flu liability, but the cost involved more than money. The stalled negotiations meant that nobody could get a shot before October 1 at the earliest. The program continued to be plagued by problems of consent forms and manufacturers' contracts and profits, but vaccine production proceeded. By October 1 the vaccinations had begun. In the meantime, both the CDC and Gallup had polled the public and estimated that 93 percent of all Americans knew about swine flu and that 53 percent intended to get the shot. But 53 percent was a long way from the stated goal of 95 percent.

On October 11 three people over the age of seventy, all with heart conditions, died in Pittsburgh, Pennsylvania, just after receiving swine flu shots at the same clinic. The media blitz began. The county suspended flu shots and nine states immediately followed suit. It took three days to sort things out and to assure the public that about a dozen people age seventy die every day in a group of 100,000. Some people would be expected to die after any event. However, the issue was still causality, and once again fear was mixed with uncertainty.

As the ultimate reassurance, members of the Ford family were televised as they received flu shots. That night, Walter Cronkite commented on his program: "The repetition of stories which appeared to link death and vaccination have spread that damage like wildfire. Hopefully it will all die down, but it will take considerable public relations efforts such as the president's well-publicized vaccination today."

The program picked up again and continued through the rest of October and into November. The results of the second field trials finally appeared. It was confirmed that children should receive two doses of the vaccine, but the vaccine inventory would allow immunizing only one child in every twelve.

By December 16 more than 40 million Americans had received shots. Never had so many people been vaccinated for the flu in one season. The number of people inoculated in different states ranged from 10 to 80 percent, reflecting perhaps that the believers in the threat of a pandemic did much more than the nonbelievers.

Through the adverse-reaction surveillance system set up by the CDC, a physician in Minnesota reported in the third week of November that one of his patients contracted Guillain-Barre Syndrome (GBS) not long after receiving a flu shot. Within a week, three more cases, one fatal, were discovered in Minnesota, followed by three others in Alabama and one in New Jersey.

Another demoralizing event had struck the struggling swine flu program. But what was even more serious was that until the risk of GBS was assessed, vaccine recipients could not be informed of it. That meant halting the program, establishing the danger of GBS, and asking for a new informed consent. After all that had happened, the virtual end of the swine flu program came because of the seriousness of a rare side effect. After nine months of labor to build defenses against an invader that never appeared, the president, with no resistance, agreed to the temporary suspension of the vaccination effort.

The new year brought a new president and a different group of legislators to Washington. For the next year there were many open hearings and meetings on influenza vaccination problems and policies. The outcome was to reconfirm the previous recommendations for vaccination of

roups, including those age sixty-five and older.
ion has resumed with the new information
ding the following statement:

> In 1976, about 12 of every 1 million adults who re-
> ceived swine influenza vaccine developed a paralytic
> condition called the Guillain-Barre Syndrome (GBS)
> within 10 weeks of vaccination. (Very little informa-
> tion is available on the risk of GBS following influ-
> enza vaccination for persons under age 18.) GBS also
> occurred in about 2 out of every 1 million adults who
> did *not* get swine influenza vaccine. Most people
> who get GBS can be expected to recover; 5–10 percent
> may have some permanent paralysis; and 5–6 percent
> may die. In 1976, there was an average of 1 death from
> GBS for every 1.8 million people vaccinated; GBS
> deaths among vaccinees over age 65 were higher—
> about 2 for every 1.8 million people vaccinated.
>
> Although most information concerning the risk of
> GBS following influenza vaccination was gathered in
> 1976, it seems likely that the risks described above
> may be present for other influenza vaccines as well.
> The risk of GBS should be balanced against the much
> higher risk of complications (including death) from
> influenza for the chronically ill and the elderly dur-
> ing influenza epidemics.

It is clear we don't know enough about the phenomenon
called influenza. We do know some things, of course, but
perhaps we have been made complacent by that knowledge long before we have enough information for effective
problem solving.

If we could go back through time to January 1976 and
have a second chance at decision making, given the same
information, what would we do? This question is not a request for second guessing, but rather a plea to extract
guidelines from the last time to help the next time. The

strategy for decision making under uncertainty is well known. Every possibility is listed, the progress of events that might follow each possibility is mapped out, and all possible outcomes of each decision recorded. To a large extent, this strategy was followed early in the swine influenza contingency planning, but we know some things now that we didn't know then. We know that antigenic shifts do not necessarily lead to pandemics and that the vaccine has some risks.

Knowing this, would the vaccine have been made at all? If so, would it have been stockpiled or given to the entire population, all those who wanted it, or only to certain target groups in the population? With the benefit of hindsight, we can now make the right decision for 1976. But what about our decision next time? It is highly unlikely that the circumstances surrounding the next potential pandemic will be precisely like those surrounding any other. Assuming, however, that a decision is made sometime in the future to undertake a massive immunization program, how will it be done?

The last element of this discussion and the theme of our book is the understanding of a complex disease. We've written many words on the antigenic changes of the virus, the short-lived effectiveness of the vaccine, the clinical confusion of many other infectious agents with the influenza virus, and our limited knowledge of the occurrence, spread, and virulence of epidemics and pandemics. These scientific issues run through and complicate every other issue about influenza. Until we possess more understanding of these scientific issues, the evidence presented to the government, public, or media will always be weak.

CHAPTER 8

How Much Will We Pay for Protection?

What is the value of a person's life? Does that value change with age? How much should society and the individual spend in attempts to prolong life? What is the cost of sickness and the price of wellness? What are the costs of changing to a preventive style of medical care? What can we afford to do and not do in meeting disease problems? How much should be spent for control of disease? The possibility of an influenza pandemic evokes all these questions. Societal apathy or fear of the next pandemic stimulates continuing debate and research on these topics.

Consider the consequences of a flu epidemic. Many older people will become ill and some will die. This loss to the community or to the nation is incalculable by any yardstick. Some businesses may fail because of the deaths of their owners; production will be sacrificed because of lost working hours; and family budgets will be strained by unexpected medical costs.

The impact of an influenza epidemic creates ever widening social and economic waves, and years later ripples may persist. Should society attempt to prevent or suppress influenza and its effects? The crass economic answer is:

Only if the cost of the disease to society is too high. An immediate retort is: But how do we calculate the cost to society? The answer is complex and elusive.

As a way of approaching the difficult questions we've posed, let's look at a basic premise of economic welfare. When people spend their money for something, the amount they will offer depends not on the future satisfaction they imagine will be realized from the thing, but on the intensity of their desire for it. Generally speaking, everybody prefers present pleasures to future pleasures of the same amount, even when there is no doubt the latter will occur.

Efforts directed toward the remote future are starved relative to efforts directed toward the present. If this economic premise is in operation, the possibility is slim that society will mount a prevention program now. An influenza immunization effort will rarely be greeted with enthusiasm. What we have described is a key stumbling block to all of preventive medicine. This quality has caused our society to be labeled a "crisis culture." We act only when we must.

Societal decisions regarding life, the quality of life, and death involve both moral and economic issues. We have only so many health resources (money, skilled workers, and supplies) to apply to our national health problems. When a decision is made to increase cancer research, possible outcomes of that decision are that more people will continue to suffer from arthritis and that there will be more deaths due to heart attacks. The problem is more complex than that, of course, and the complexity generally shields the decision-maker from any moral concern.

Implicit in societal concern for life and death are two questions: what is the value of a person's life and how much ought society (including the person) spend in attempts to prolong it? From these questions we can construct the following statement: If society could be sure that the costs of efforts to preserve a person's life *now* would be equal to the *future* worth of the individual's life, then the decision to preserve could be based on moral issues. Such a pronouncement asserts that it is not appropriate for the economist to assign objective values now to the fear, suffering, and damage people experience because of a serious illness in the future. Consider a nonmedical example. A school board may be faced with deciding how much of its budget to spend on school bus safety, knowing that every additional dollar spent on bus monitors' and drivers' salaries will reduce the quality of education by a certain amount. Presumably the school board represents the preferences of the public and is capable of making this decision. Often, however, the money allocated to safety is in a multiuse fund, and there is no way to avoid, at least implicitly, placing a dollar value on safety. And that is the question. How should society go about placing a dollar value on the health and safety effects of a public program?

We speculate that most of our citizens are interested not only in prolonging their lives but also in living their lives under conditions of reduced risk. The avoidance of sickness or death from influenza is not like usual choices or actions. It involves anxiety, sentiment, knowledge, guilt, awe, responsibility, and religion. Whether one deals with an individual or a societal group, manifestations of these conditions can be detected.

Suppose an influenza immunization program intended to reduce sickness and save lives is proposed, and we want to know its worth. Assume that a large known population is likely to be attacked by the virus. We are aware of what the risk is and have a good idea of how much reduction of risk we can achieve. Moreover, unless we expect an invasion of something like the 1918 strain of virus, we generally expect the risk to be relatively small, and not a serious source of anxiety or guilt.

If we can collect the cost of the immunization program

from the people who stand to benefit from it, surely these beneficiaries should be allowed to have the program. To determine if the economic benefits are worth the costs, we need to know what people will pay for the program.

The trouble with asking people what they think the program is worth is that most individuals are unable to answer hypothetical questions about important events. A case of the flu and its accompanying minor risk of death requires that a person deal with the minute probability that an awesome event will happen, and no amount of intellect, imagination, or analogy may reveal what avoiding the event is worth. Death is not something we practice. Most of us think about it only when we witness the sorrow of a friend, experience serious illness, or write a will. Not only are the consumers of vaccinations poor at making choices about anything related to death, but they will evade these questions given a chance.

In the case of an influenza vaccination program, it is likely to turn out that some consumers have a strong interest, others a weak interest, and still others will oppose the program. People will be concerned if the price of the program is high or if the tax system does not distribute the costs where the benefits fall. Some consumers may cite the "pricelessness of human life" as a basis for decision making, but we should not think it strange that the rich will pay more for longevity than the poor, and the rich prefer programs that help the rich and the poor those that help the poor.

What we have been describing is in accord with a basic principle of welfare economics, that is, measure program benefit as the sum of all affected individuals' willingness to pay for the proposed program. In the case of flu vaccination, it might work something like this. Each household would be informed of how a proposed flu vaccination program might influence the safety of the family members, and each household would be asked to return a ballot on which they indicate the maximum amount they would be willing to pay to have the program enacted. Answers would reflect financial circumstances and how much risk reduction persons seek. If the sum of the family contributions exceeds the cost of the vaccination program, presumably we should go ahead with the program.

One obvious practical problem is that developing accurate assessments of an individual's willingness to pay is difficult, expensive, and time consuming. Two approaches have been used. By studying a household carefully and observing the implicit value placed on safety and health in consumption and job selection, inferences are made regarding how much the household values mortality reduction. The second, more direct method uses survey questionnaires that ask heads of households to state their willingness to pay for the program benefit that is under consideration.

Implicit willingness to pay for lifesaving measures can be inferred from the higher wages paid in occupations with above-average risk of death. Unfortunately, however, to be included in this measurement a person must be working for wages, and that excludes housewives, children, retired people, and others who are not paid for their work. Even more complicated questions emerge when we try to compare the wages of a race car driver with those of a taxi driver, questions like: Are we considering representative people? Is there a prestige payoff beyond the dollars received, and can it be estimated? Were wages accepted at the outset truly indicative of the danger involved? Using this approach, one investigator inferred a value of between $176,000 and $260,000 per life saved.

The inferences of the previous paragraph are difficult to make and are likely to be error-laden. If we are trying to find a proxy measure for people's willingness to pay for risk aversion, why not just ask them? Studies designed to determine willingness to pay revealed what you might suspect. A person's willingness to pay increases with increasing probability of death and when greater reductions of risk are offered by the program.

Let's turn the question of the willingness to pay now, in order to avoid future risk, inside out. Ask the consumer how much payment will be demanded now in order to run some additional risk in the future. Might he or she prefer to run the risk and put the proceeds in an investment? These questions raise the uncomfortable issue of how much monetary compensation a family needs in order to experience no long-term loss in welfare when a member of the family dies. Is it surprising that while a family would not give up all its income to save one member, this same family would reject as inadequate any economic compensation?

Society's uncertainty about mounting an influenza vaccination program stems not from the problem of evaluating the worth of a person's livelihood to the different people who have an interest in it, but from the worth of that person's life to himself or herself or to whoever will pay to prolong it. It is possible to charge each program beneficiary less than his or her share if a "cost benefit" viewpoint is taken. This attitude recognizes that lives saved and illnesses avoided benefit society as well as the individuals involved. Here too there is a trade-off between dollars and mortality rates, and there is plenty of precedence for making that balance as we've described.

There is significant importance in society's maintaining a public commitment to the preservation of life. This commitment is part of the foundation of a stable society. Nevertheless, how public money is to be divided between protecting a group of elderly people from an influenza epidemic and protecting a group of coal miners from the inadequate safety practices of their employers is a complex issue. In both cases, people will die without government intervention.

We might suspect that society is not concerned about the particular cause of death that a program attempts to curtail. What counts is the number and possibly the characteristics of lives saved. Estimate some "value of life," multiply it by the number of lives saved, and the result will be the societal benefit of the program. However, if public safety programs are evaluated from this viewpoint, no consistency of result is found. A few thousand dollars is required to save one life in a highway design, while in excess of a million dollars is necessary to protect the pilot in a bomber. The excessive variation in the cost of safety in airplanes compared to cars is often substantiated by the greater anxiety air passengers experience about a crash, even though their probabilistic risk is lower.

A more dispassionate look at the cost of public safety will reveal that most of the variation is caused by complicated decision-making processes, special political interests, and ignorance. A person's potential earnings for the remainder of his or her life are often taken as an indicator of what he or she would spend to increase the likelihood of survival. Discounting lifetime earnings may be relevant for ordinary consumption, but what an individual would pay to avoid sickness, to avoid death, or to acquire a racing sailboat bears no simple relationship. In addition, there is no reason to believe that changes in earnings have any obvious relationship to what society values in health or safety program outcomes.

It's easy to consult a table to determine incomes of persons of different ages according to sex, race, and education. Numbers, especially in tabular form, have a disproportionate influence on many people. But controversial assumptions underlie any future earnings table. If, for example, a decision-maker saw a treatment of housewives' activities in a table, instant rejection of the data becomes a strong possibility.

Anxiety about impending danger may give no impetus

to the vaccination program. Most consumers who take a close look at their own anxieties recognize a controllable psychological phenomenon. The cause and amount of risk influence the sense of anxiety. Very low levels of risk may be ignored and high levels may become an obsession.

As difficult as it is to determine costs in a cost-benefit study of an influenza vaccination program, the benefits are infinitely more difficult to calculate. Lifetime earnings are usually involved, and these figures must take into account life expectancy for different age, sex, and racial groups, how long a working life is, changing patterns of earnings at successive ages, the value of housewives' services, and any change in the value of money over time.

A possible source of misunderstanding about cost-benefit analysis is that direct benefits are usually costs presently borne that would be averted if the health program in question proved to be effective. These costs must be separated from the resource costs required to conduct that program.

Direct benefits represent potential tangible savings in the use of health resources. When two diseases are present in a patient, the issues become complicated. The presence of the second disease often changes the costs of intervention and therefore the direct benefits. Gains in future earnings, a part of indirect benefits, are also affected because the presence of the second disease influences the recovery from the first.

Economists, drawing on the data resources of both the federal government and unpublished sources, have tabulated their estimates of lost earnings. Earnings never to be received because of sickness and death can be found in the long columns.

Let's take a different tack on these treacherous seas. Think of health as an investment. The concept of health is a complex, elusive subject, so let's substitute the word *wellness* for health. How much will an individual pay to sustain wellness? A person is more effective in society both as a producer and as a consumer when in a state of wellness. We can use simple arithmetic to compute income changes due to illness and death, but what would be the loss to the Western world if Einstein had died during the flu epidemic following World War I?

Anyone investing in his or her own wellness would like to be sure that the money spent will affect the state of wellness. Given our present understanding, it is difficult to disentangle the effects on the population that are attributable to health programs from those influenced by better nutrition, improved housing, better working conditions, and higher incomes.

In the past, some cultures made a larger investment in health by killing the disabled and weak in order to raise the health status of the culture. Biological selection is no longer an acceptable method of investing in health, not only because our humanitarian sensibilities reject it, but also because it costs too much. To some extent our investment in health improves the labor product and continues to provide a return over several years. This human capital formation by health care has been measured in various ways. If we evaluate the cost of health care of people currently in the labor force, we can then ask about the money value of the annual labor product that is added as a consequence of the health investments made.

Calculations exist in which a summation of the following items has been done: medical care costs of childbearing, health costs for an infant and child, and medical care expenditures for a child up to age eighteen. Such a computation gives the health care costs of producing a labor force member aged eighteen. These people may be valued at the present value of future earnings generated through the health programs. A crass economic view, to be sure, but there's more. Next, as a means of determining the value of the health care delivered, the expected return on the investment is calculated.

Assume we mounted a prevention program and as a result society gained a human labor resource. Two questions are asked: How much would those people who are now sick have produced? As for those who were prevented from getting sick, how much will they add to national income?

A rough estimate of the national gain attributable to the prevention of sickness and death can be made by adding up the economic effects of the deaths of workers, the loss of working time, and the loss of productive capacity while at work. The calculation is simple: Estimate the gain in productive work time and multiply by a suitable per unit time money value.

However, what we've described is anything but simple. For example, if unemployment exists, the prevention program may enlarge the percent of people out of work. Adding to the complexity is the fact that unemployment, with its emotional and physical impacts, will increase the incidence of illness.

The assumption that people saved from the ravages of one disease are available for national gain is also false. It is possible that persons saved from one disease may promptly die of another. Especially among older people, the treatment required to overcome one disease weakens an individual and he or she is more prone to other ailments.

Collecting data that honor the division between disability (staying home) and debility (working, but poorly) is difficult. In our culture there are some blind people who are considered disabled and are excluded from the work force, others who have sheltered employment with limited output, and still others who, as scientists, writers, or in other skilled professions, make significant contributions and reflect neither disability nor debility. The loss of working efficiency is no simple matter to define and measure. People silently experience the full range of good to bad days, and the impact on functioning may be subtle.

If all the difficulties we've cited can be overcome, and if the number of productive man-years added because of the prevention program can be calculated, this information may prove a useful political tool. The real political power, however, lies in translating it into dollars gained.

Two approaches have been used to assign a dollar value to each unit of labor work time. The first approach divides the value of all things produced by the number of workers who produced them. The average dollar value of each unit of labor work time is used to forecast the gains of the larger labor force. In the second approach, average earnings are multiplied by the number of man-years added as a result of the prevention of disease. The result is a dollar estimate of the national gain. Whichever approach is used, the result is an estimate of the dollar value of the labor lost as a consequence of death, disability, and debility. The prevention or cure of these conditions gives an estimate of added income.

It's all a complex economic trade-off. Health programs use skilled people and materials to create economic resources. In this analysis the humanitarian aspects are, of course, excluded.

In recent times, consumer preferences have been used as a guide for the best use of health resources. But the consumer's preferences for work, leisure, and income are not simply applied in the "health marketplace." If a person is vaccinated against an infectious disease his or her neighbors who make no purchases of vaccine also benefit. Thus the social value of medical services is often much larger than the private value to those making the investment in

themselves. Other medical services obviously outside the
price market system include water pollution control, fluo-
ridation of water supplies, and mosquito control. The marketplace viewpoint is further limited by the fact that our
health resources are allocated by a complex combination
of both private market and administrative decisions.

Individual behavior regarding influenza contains three
aspects. First, all manner of upper respiratory disease is
referred to as "flu," which supports the notion that people
are aware of influenza and expect a bout now and then,
even though their understanding of the disease is imprecise. Second, a substantial majority of people do not view
themselves as susceptible to the most serious effects of influenza. Third, there is a widespread lack of concern about
the severity of the disease.

The behavior we've just described functions within a
general awareness that a vaccine is not an absolute means
of controlling a disease. There is no doubt that this behavior has contributed to a general lack of success of carrying
out a national influenza vaccine policy.

Four compelling reasons exist for developing and im-
plementing positive measures to control epidemic influenza. First, though the disease is generally benign, epidemics are usually accompanied by excess mortality.
Many of the people who die were not at death's door when
influenza struck. Second, influenza can strike so many
people in such a short time that the epidemic is quite capable of interrupting the orderly flow of community life. Excessive absenteeism can cripple police, fire, transportation, telephone, and medical services. Third, the costs of
epidemic influenza to society can run into billions of dollars per outbreak. The cost can reach staggering levels by
any standard, but particularly in comparison with the
costs of other acute infectious diseases.

And finally, exposure to influenza does not guarantee

anything approaching lasting immunity. Virtually the entire population must be considered at risk of infection from either a new virus or a different form of a virus already experienced. Even though older people have a lower risk of infection, this is more than offset by the peril of complications and the increase in death rates.

In one study an estimate was made of the costs of epidemic influenza from October 1968 to March 1969. The study included direct costs, such as expenditures for physicians' services, hospital stays, and prescription costs, and indirect costs that reflected the productivity temporarily foregone due to sickness or permanently lost due to death.

The total direct cost based on 21,332,000 physician visits was estimated at $637,104,000. The national economic loss due to deaths was $1,287,791,000; that due to sickness, $1,955,135,000. Therefore, during the 1968–69 epidemic when 27,495 people died, the total cost was estimated at just under $4 billion. Manipulating these or other statistics might be impressive to some readers, but we believe that these numbers for one "routine" epidemic need no embellishment.

The disease prevention offered by well-conceived and efficiently delivered influenza immunization programs can contribute to prolonging life expectancy. While we can comfortably predict some longevity gains, it is not at all clear that reducing this major cause of sickness and death can reduce the costs of disease care. People are in effect being "saved" for many competing causes of sickness and death that strike in old age.

Society, with its current social, legislative, and economic rules, is beginning to realize that a successful disease-prevention program has diminishing economic benefit as more people reach and live well beyond retirement age. In fact, if the potential benefits of influenza vaccination of the elderly are reduced to pure economic terms we must also consider the costs of saving many lives that may be economic ''burdens.'' Fortunately, we haven't become that calloused. We feel confident that our society will continue to make the requisite changes in social and economic policies to foster longer and healthier lives.

CHAPTER 9

To Be Shot, or Not?

All of us in the past few years have read articles with headlines like these: "SENATE APPROVES PROPOSAL FOR FREE INFLUENZA SHOTS," "ARE WE HEADED FOR ANOTHER FLU FIASCO?" "FLU VACCINES, THEY ARE AT IT AGAIN," "THE LINGERING EFFECTS OF SWINE FLU," "SWINE FLU SCARE," "JUDGE REJECTS GOVERNMENT RULE ON COMPENSATION OVER FLU SHOTS," "ORIGINS OF RUSSIAN INFLUENZA," and finally, "SWINE FLU CLAIMS TOTAL NEARLY $900 MILLION."

Vaccines for smallpox, polio, measles, rubella, and mumps have attracted no such brickbats. In fact, today's newspaper stories are more likely to describe "miracle" vaccines. It is something of a miracle that a potion devised by man has defeated the ancient enemy, smallpox. No naturally occurring cases of smallpox have been detected since October 26, 1977, in Merko, Somalia.

In the developed countries, polio is no longer considered the dread crippler. The only naturally occurring cases of polio remaining in the developed nations involve immigrants from less-developed countries or people who refuse vaccination for personal reasons. Today, there are

ɔlio cases per year. Some of these cases
vaccine itself. However, concern over
ɪssociated case of polio has not resulted
ɔ ban the vaccine. The benefits of the vac-
recognized as outweighing the risks.

ɪe of vaccination, measles and its fellow travelers ɔ. ɪalitis, pneumonia, and deafness have decreased dramatically. Since approval for the use of live
measles virus vaccine in 1963, the number of cases of measles in the United States has been cut back from nearly
500,000 cases per year to about 3,000 in 1981. Measles can
still strike among our children whose parents neglect to
have them vaccinated, and the press has strongly ap-
plauded the government's efforts to increase measles immunization among children who receive no regular medical care.

Few question the use of rubella vaccine to prevent the
infection of pregnant women and its tragic impact on the
unborn child—deafness, blindness, deformity, and men-
tal retardation. Vaccination is recommended for all children, even though except for experiencing a mild rash and
a slight fever, most youngsters are hardly aware of the disease. Although some ethical questions crop up regarding
the rights of the male vaccinee versus the public health
needs of society, most physicians find no conflict in vacci-
nating males in order to decrease the spread of the disease
to mothers who have not been immunized. There has been
no outburst in the news media or in the halls of Congress,
in spite of the theoretical and controversial nature of this
practice. The incidence of rubella has decreased dramatically.

Finally, although it is less strongly recommended for
general public immunization, mumps vaccine is well accepted by pediatricians as a safe and effective method of
preventing this disease. Serious consequences of mumps

during childhood are rare, but most parents take advantage of the vaccine to prevent their children from having swollen jaws or their sons from suffering the more serious complication of orchitis later in life. There is no controversy here. The number of cases continues to go down.

Why, then, is there so much fuss over the flu vaccine? A poll commissioned by the government in early December 1976, during the final weeks of the swine flu immunization program, revealed that over 90 percent of its respondents were aware of the immunization program and that most even knew where to obtain the shots. However, awareness and good intent are not synonymous with action. Only 32 percent had actually had the vaccine. Of interest are the main answers of those who said they were not planning to be immunized. Over one-third said they did not feel the shots were necessary. Slightly less than one-third said they feared the pain of the shots. Ten percent felt the shots would do no good. These findings may or may not hold true today, but it would be useful to examine some of the facts regarding the vaccine that may bear on the public's perception.

Each year in late January or February, WHO publishes formal recommendations regarding the virus strains that should be included in the vaccine for the next season. These judgments are based on which strains are currently in circulation, how long they have been around, how different they are antigenically from current vaccine strains, and the size of the outbreaks or epidemics reported for each strain.

This information must be issued nearly a year in advance, and often before the influenza season in the Northern Hemisphere is underway. Manufacturers need the lead time to produce and distribute the vaccine. In spite of great care and careful predictions, new strains may unexpectedly appear in the spring and become dominant. By then it is usually too late to change the vaccine, and it must be used as is, with the hope that the same strain will continue during the next season.

Neither the United States nor any other nation is obligated to use the WHO recommendations. Through the influenza center in Atlanta and the *Weekly Epidemiologic Record*, the United States has access to the same information utilized by WHO. In practice, however, since we participate in the WHO decision-making process, WHO's recommendations and ours tend to be the same, although there have been some exceptions.

Vaccine formulation, potency, purity, and safety are the responsibility in the United States of the Bureau of Biologics (BoB) of the FDA. Decisions for the next flu season are made with the assistance of outside advisors, appropriate representatives, the CDC, the NIH, the armed forces, and the manufacturers. Recommendations on vaccine formulation and dosage are usually made in January or February.

The CDC and its Advisory Committee on Immunization Practices (ACIP) recommend who should receive the vaccine. This group usually meets in early spring to announce its recommendations for the coming flu season. ACIP members are epidemiologists, pediatricians, and others chosen from the staffs of county and state health departments and schools of public health. Also attending these meetings are representatives from BoB, NIH, the armed forces, the American Academy of Pediatrics committee on infectious diseases, and other experts, including representatives from other countries. Both the BoB and the ACIP meetings are open and are often attended by members of the news media. Recommendations of the ACIP on influenza vaccinations are printed in July in the *Weekly Morbidity and Mortality Report*, published by CDC.

Unlike polio, measles, rubella, or mumps vaccines, which use the same virus stock every year, influenza vaccines are changed frequently, causing new production headaches nearly every year. Complicating the production problems even more is the fact that there are four American flu vaccine manufacturers, Parke-Davis, Wyeth, Connaught, and Merck, Sharp and Dohme, each with a different manufacturing process and different virus growth requirements. These companies begin to worry in December, and in January they are openly concerned about the vaccine they must produce.

In most years, however, when a change in the vaccine is expected, the manufacturers receive candidate strains in order to begin to raise "breeding stock" for their vaccine as early as possible. These strains are the offspring from "marrying" a new virus strain to an established vaccine strain to produce a virus that has the antigenic characteristics of the new strain and the growth characteristics of an established strain. In this way it is possible to accelerate vaccine production.

All manufacturers grow the vaccine virus in hens' eggs. Millions of eggs containing live ten- to eleven-day-old embryos are injected with several hundred virus "breeding stock" particles each. The embryos are kept at body temperature or slightly below for forty-eight hours to allow the viruses to multiply. Later, when the tops of the eggs are removed and the whitish egg fluid is collected, each egg yields tens of millions of viruses. The virus is then concentrated, purified, killed by the addition of formaldehyde, diluted to proper strength, and bottled for distribution.

Some manufacturers produce "whole" vaccines of purified, intact virus particles, and others produce "split" vaccines of purified virus particles that have been disrupted by various chemical procedures. The technical details of each process are trade secrets, but regardless of the methods used, each manufacturer meets the same federal requirements for vaccine purity and potency. Vaccines are

drugs and are under the control of the FDA. Each manufacturer is licensed and must undergo periodic inspection of
production facilities and batch-by-batch evaluation of vaccines.

A major problem is determining the required vaccine
potency standards. The problems are technical and complex but hinge on these two facts: the killed vaccine contains more than one virus type and is prepared by different
methods by several manufacturers. Potency standards for
measles vaccine are easier to establish. They require that
an accepted attenuated vaccine strain be used and that the
final product contain a certain number of live virus particles. In the case of the flu vaccine, the same strain is not
used every year; also it may contain two strains of influenza A and one strain of B. The number of live particles
cannot be measured because the virus is dead. Influenza
vaccine potency standards rely heavily on sensitive laboratory tests to determine the precise amount of the specific
component of the virus necessary for immunity.

There have been two large-scale field trials of influenza
vaccines in recent times: The 1976 swine flu vaccine trials
used over seven thousand volunteers, and the 1978 Russian flu vaccine trials used more than twenty-five hundred
volunteers. People of different ages who have been exposed to different flu viruses over the years behave immu-
nologically quite differently. Whether the vaccine is split
or whole is much less important than the individual's
"original antigenic sin." Persons born before 1957 and infected with influenza viruses at some time during their
lives readily produced antibody to the swine flu virus, but
those born after 1957 did not. For the second group, two
doses of vaccine, spaced at least four weeks apart, were required to achieve the same immunity as the first group.

The different individual responses to vaccine create
enormous headaches for public health personnel. Testing
produces a myriad of recommendations that, although

necessary, can complicate any vaccination program. For example, during the swine flu vaccine program one dose of split or whole vaccine was adequate for those over twenty-four years of age. Two doses were required for those twenty-three and under. For those below age twelve, only split virus could be used, and fractions of adult doses were required. There were split virus vaccines, whole virus vaccines, vaccines containing only swine flu, vaccines containing two type A strains, and even a type B strain of vaccine was available. Little wonder the public was confused.

We have learned a great deal about vaccine potency standards during the past few years. New tests minimize the discrepancies between whole and split vaccines. Since it is not possible to conduct time-consuming and expensive field trials with volunteers before each change in vaccine formulation, we must count on laboratory tests as the primary means for evaluating vaccine potency.

Veterans of military service during the 1950s and 1960s remember the sore arms and fever after flu shots. Some insisted they had the flu only after they received the vaccine. The flu shots weren't the only shots that hurt—so did the vaccines against typhus, typhoid, cholera, Japanese B encephalitis, and spotted fever. In fact, most people who received the early Rocky Mountain spotted fever vaccine were convinced that it still contained the rocks. Vaccines have come a long way since then. Typhus, typhoid, and cholera vaccines still hurt, but immediate discomfort caused by influenza vaccines is much less, thanks largely to improved vaccine purification methods since 1969. During the swine flu trials, less than 2 percent of adults who received the program vaccine were feverish. Split vaccines caused immediate reactions less often than whole vaccines. In the 1978 trials, even with the maximum dose of vaccine, less than 4 percent of the people felt malaise, headache, and fever. We can't do much better than that. Even the pure virus has some toxic properties.

Of course, "safe" vaccine does not refer to sore arms and fever occurring up to forty-eight hours after injection. We are concerned primarily about the more serious, often delayed, adverse reactions. Just prior to the swine flu immunization program, a thorough search of the medical literature revealed that during the previous thirty years of influenza vaccination in the United States, there were nine reported cases of neurological illnesses following injection. All of the patients recovered. Whether or not the illnesses were caused by the vaccine is uncertain. There were three reports of death following influenza vaccination. The most recent report in 1963 described neurological complication and death of a fifteen-year-old diabetic four days after receiving the vaccine. In 1947, a three-year-old girl ran a temperature of 109 degrees and died four hours after receiving the vaccine. The earliest report described an army recruit who received influenza, typhus, and cholera vaccines simultaneously. He died thirty minutes after receiving all three vaccines.

The flu vaccine after-effect statistics changed when the swine flu vaccine campaign was well underway. By late November and early December 1976, about two months after the program began, cases of Guillain-Barre Syndrome (GBS) were reported through the surveillance program designed to monitor vaccine reactions. The vaccinations were stopped on December 16 to assess the extent of GBS and its possible connection to the vaccine.

GBS is not a new disease brought on only by the vaccine. It is a rare disease that has been attributed to many different causes. The major source of concern was that the occurrence among vaccinees was about ten times that among nonvaccinees, or about one case per 100,000 vaccinees. The risk of GBS among vaccinees was lowest in children and highest among those over twenty-five years old. GBS was fatal in one case among about 2 million vaccinees.

Our concern about the link between GBS and influenza vaccinees is not shared by other countries with similar vaccine practices and products. In Japan, for example, by law nearly 18 million schoolchildren are given inactivated influenza vaccine each year. An additional 3 million or so adults receive the vaccine annually. Japan reports no evidence of vaccine-related GBS. Because of its rarity, it conceivably could be overlooked in adults, but not in children, in whose cases better records are kept. We do not know why GBS appeared in specimens in the United States but not in Japan. One speculation suggests genetic predisposition to GBS in the United States. Another possible explanation is that GBS appears less frequently among younger vaccinees. Another conjectures that GBS is associated only with the swine flu vaccine, which was never used in Japan. Support for the latter comes from the national GBS surveillance program conducted by the Center for Disease Control. Vaccines used in the four years since the swine flu program have not been statistically associated with increases in GBS. GBS may not be a risk with every influenza vaccine, but we must assume it might be until proven otherwise.

Hardly anyone outside of the medical profession knew of GBS prior to the swine flu program. Now it's a household world. GBS is classified as an ascending paralysis, that is, some numbness and paralysis is often noted first in the feet. Paralysis will either spread no further or spread inconsistently over days or weeks to involve legs, hands, arms, and, in fatal cases, the muscles that assist in breathing. GBS is thought to be an "autoimmune" disease. Cells in the patient's immunologic system go wild and attack the substance covering the nerves. As a consequence, the nerves are short-circuited, and no messages, or only confused messages, get through. Usually the patient recovers both feeling and movement when a new nerve covering grows back. The cause of this damage is not known. Possi-

bly certain people are susceptible to GBS and at critical
times in their lives any shock, including vaccines, to their
immunologic system serves to trigger it. We don't know
how to identify such people.

General allergic reactions to influenza vaccines are even
more rare than GBS. During the swine flu program only
one such reaction occurred in about 4 million shots. No
one died. It is extremely difficult to prove that any rarely
occurring reaction is caused by a specific drug or vaccine.
By chance alone, someone has a heart attack after going to
the grocery store, after returning from work, or after taking
a flu shot. It is not enough that "something" rare happens
following an event, but rather that "something" must follow the same event more frequently than expected. In
other words, the number of times that the event occurs
must be larger than just chance alone. An episode preced-
ing a rare event is not necessarily the cause of the event.

To answer the question, "Is the vaccine safe?" we can
answer yes for 99,999 of 100,000 people. Is this good
enough?

The value of a drug or vaccine is determined by more
than simply "nine out of ten doctors prescribe it" or by
your trust in it. Impressions or opinions have no place in
science. To prove that a drug or vaccine is safe and effective requires extensive study under carefully controlled
test conditions. Typically, one large group receives the
medication being tested and another large group receives
an inert substance made to resemble the drug as much as
possible. Neither the volunteer nor the physician knows
which is the product and which is the placebo. In this way,
neither the volunteer nor the physician is likely to show
bias in reporting side effects or the beneficial effects of the
drug. Only when the test is complete and the results studied can it be known whether or not the drug works.

Paradoxically, at a time when the public is asking for

more proof of the usefulness of drugs, it is less willing to volunteer for vaccine trials or for any test that involves a risk, real or imagined. This resistance to helping with medical research makes scientific proof expensive and difficult to achieve.

There have been many field trials of influenza vaccines. The ideal trials are those that determine influenza vaccine efficacy; that is, how well does the vaccine prevent disease? Hundreds of healthy volunteers are required for such studies; volunteers who won't get very sick, if infected, and who are willing to gamble on receiving either the vaccine or a placebo. Many field tests are initiated, but few succeed. Either no flu appears that year, the attack rate is too small, the flu arrives just as the study gets underway, or it is the wrong type of flu! The potential pitfalls are many. Even if the efficacy trials are underway and flu does arrive on time, proving that the shot kept a person well is not easy.

Several years ago a sportswriter with a sense of humor set out to prove that his local small college (we shall call it Podunk) football team, loser in every game but one, was actually better than that year's national champion, which won every game but one. He did this by showing that the one game won by Podunk College was an upset against team B, which had, in turn, beaten team G, which had beaten team P, and so on, until team X had finally upset the national champions in their one defeat. Sometimes it seems that proponents and opponents of flu vaccine play the same game—but without tongue-in-cheek. Anyone can use field trial results to support any point of view. This is hardly reassuring and certainly not in keeping with the lofty ideals of science. To understand this, let's examine the variables that influence a vaccine efficacy trial.

The basic formula for calculating vaccine efficacy is simple and can be written as:

$$\frac{\left(\begin{array}{c}\text{No. cases influenza} \\ \text{in placebo group}\end{array}\right) \text{ minus } \left(\begin{array}{c}\text{No. cases influenza} \\ \text{in vaccine group}\end{array}\right)}{\text{No. cases influenza in placebo group}} \times 100$$

The result is the percentage protection given by the vaccine. This formula for vaccine efficacy works well for measles or polio, for example, where the clinical diagnosis is simple and objective. It is too elementary for influenza, since clinical diagnosis is highly subjective and may be confused with respiratory illness caused by other agents.

Several different methods have been proposed to make efficacy figures for influenza vaccine more meaningful. The simplest is to count as cases only those persons with laboratory-proven influenza. That is, the illness is diagnosed either by virus isolation or by evidence of an antibody increase (to the epidemic strain) from acute to convalescent blood specimens. Isolation of the virus for every patient is a big job. Therefore, most trials depend on antibody increases for diagnosis. The objectors to this approach insist that persons with vaccine-induced antibody may later have the disease but show no further antibody rise. Such people are not scored as cases, making the vaccine look better than it really is. To overcome this objection, another method adjusts the clinical attack rate for influenzalike illness in the vaccine group for the laboratory-proven influenza attack rate in the placebo group. The trouble with this tactic is that it doesn't take into account any increased incidence of noninfluenza disease in the vaccine group; therefore, it makes the vaccine look worse than it really is. To illustrate the variation in vaccine efficacy rates obtained by these three methods, look at the results of four well-controlled field trials conducted during the Hong Kong epidemic of 1968–69.

There is plenty to argue about here. During the same epidemic, with the same virus, the clinical protection rate ranged from 0 to 62 percent, the adjusted rate from 25 to 77 percent, and the laboratory rate from 86 to 90 percent. What was the protection?

Trial No.	Percentage Protection (Vaccine Efficacy)		
	Clinical	Laboratory	Adjusted Laboratory
1	0	Not done	90
2	20	25	88
3	44	78	86
4	62	77	88

The most consistent findings of influenza vaccine protection have been reported by the army's commission on influenza. In twenty-five years of conducting vaccine trials in the military, this group found protection rates that ranged from 67 to 90 percent for influenza A. Such rates, however, are calculated from laboratory-proven cases, which in the military are generally based on more strict criteria for the diagnosis of influenza than are usually found in most civilian studies. When civilian studies consider bed confinement as a disease criterion, vaccine protection rates soar. This may mean that the vaccine ameliorates the disease even if it doesn't fully prevent it or that it is more difficult to separate mild influenza from background respiratory disease. It is probably both.

Occasionally vaccine failures are reported in both civilian and military groups. An obvious failure occurs when the vaccine prepared in the spring does not contain the virus that unexpectedly appears the next fall or winter. Such viruses show antigenic shift (as in 1957, 1968, and 1977) or more commonly antigenic drift. If shift is involved, the vaccine is useless. If drift occurs, vaccine protection rates are likely to be reduced, depending on the magnitude of drift.

From 1969 through 1977, the virus strains used in the vaccine were identical for four of the years to the strain(s) that caused disease. For four years they contained closely related but not identical strains. During the 1977–78 season, four strains caused illness. The strains in the vaccines were closely related to two of them, less well related to a third (because of drift), and not at all related to the fourth (because of shift).

The flu season would be over each year before protection trials could be completed for every flu vaccine. The scientific community accepts antibody response data in lieu of evidence that the vaccine would prevent flu caused by that virus. Protection given by a vaccine is estimated by the frequency and amount of antibody stimulated in volunteers. There is clearly a difference, however, between achieving a certain level of antibody through vaccination alone and achieving that same level through natural disease or by boosting naturally acquired antibody through vaccination. Naturally acquired protection probably involves other immunity mechanisms. Only large field studies are likely to give some of the answers to these questions.

How long-lasting is the protection offered by vaccination? Annual vaccination is recommended, but some protection has been reported to last up to three years. Again, it is critical to separate the people whose antibody levels have been boosted through vaccination and those who have achieved antibody for the first time through vaccination. In the second group, antibody levels are known to decrease after three months.

In summary, does the vaccine work? There is general agreement that when the vaccine contains the most current virus strains at the proper strengths, it provides protection or ameliorates illness caused by the influenza virus. There is considerably less agreement on how much protection the vaccine affords. And there is no consensus on the beneficial long-term effects of annual vaccination. More study is essential.

Influenza vaccine isn't used to control the disease. It is a way of providing individual protection. Except for 1976, when it was recommended that the general population receive the vaccine, the emphasis has been on an annual offering of vaccine to people most likely to experience serious illness or death from influenza. The vaccine is always available to a physician for any person needing and wanting it. There are no restrictions on its use. Nevertheless, the annual recommendations receive a mixed response. Many want to see the vaccine recommended for everyone, particularly for children, and others want to see it recommended for no one.

Criticism is often aimed at the federal government for making recommendations but having no policy for delivery of the vaccine. Several states have had modest programs for providing vaccines to high-risk persons. Except for the swine flu program, 1978 was the first time the federal government supplied vaccine to participating states and helped pay for the vaccinations. This vaccine was intended for only the high-risk groups.

The $8.2 million allotted to the vaccine grants program for 1978 was adequate to provide vaccine for a little over 3 million people. More than 42 million of our citizens are considered in danger from influenza. About 20 percent of this high-risk group receives shots now—mainly from private physicians. The federal program in 1978 called for a gradual increase in annual support to individual states until everyone in the high-risk group who wanted a flu shot could have it. The federal program was discontinued in 1980. Some state and local governments continued publicly supported influenza vaccination programs through 1981, but the numbers of such programs have continued to dwindle because of lack of funds.

The obvious benefit of using influenza vaccines is a reduction in the risks of becoming ill and of dying from influenza. It has been estimated that in 1968 people over sixty-five had about one chance in ten of catching A/Hong Kong flu. Once infected, they had nearly one chance in fifty of dying. This is in contrast to the one chance in a million or greater of dying from a vaccine-associated reaction such as GBS. On statistical grounds, the odds are obviously in favor of the vaccines as long as they provide protection.

No controlled study has been done, or ever will be done, to prove the effectiveness of the vaccine in preventing death. We cannot conduct an experiment where death is the end point. However, we can use a little arithmetic to calculate the theoretical risks and benefits that accrue to the nation as a result of vaccination. In 1968, for example, the influenza attack rate for people over sixty-five was about 10 percent, a bit lower than usual. Estimating 40 million persons age sixty-five or older, we list 4 million elderly people as ill with influenza during that winter season. Excess mortality during that epidemic was about 33,000, and 80 percent of the deaths occurred among the elderly; therefore, 26,000 excess deaths occurred among those sixty-five years of age or older. If all 40 million elderly persons had been vaccinated prior to the epidemic and if the vaccine had been at least 70 percent effective, then possibly 18,000 lives would have been saved. This is simply an estimate, of course. But this estimate would be supported by at least one study conducted in 1972 by a group in Seattle. They showed that vaccination of the elderly members of a prepaid health plan was associated with an estimated 72 percent reduction in hospitalization and an 87 percent reduction in deaths.

Compare this with the risk figures for GBS. There are 11 to 16 naturally occurring cases of GBS per million persons per year. Swine flu-related GBS cases were 4.5 per million vaccinees age eighteen to twenty-four and 10 per million vaccinees age fifty and above. We've said that the vaccine may be simply one more triggering mechanism for people who are predisposed to GBS. The crucial point, however, is that a person has no choice about whether a naturally occurring disease may trigger GBS, but he or she does have a choice in electing to take the vaccine. To put the relative risks of GBS into perspective, a person is 10,000 times more likely to die from a simple appendectomy, a woman is 5,000 times more likely to die following an elective hysterectomy, and one is 160 to 600 times more likely to die from an adverse reaction to penicillin. The immunization of 40 million elderly persons may have caused 400 cases of GBS, which could result in 20 deaths. This number is much smaller than the 18,000 deaths that might have resulted from influenza.

This analysis serves the public health point of view, but the arithmetic may be a little too simple and the data based on too many assumptions. First, we assume that the vaccine protection offered the young and healthy is the same as that given the elderly. This isn't necessarily true. Second, we assume that the excess mortality figures are reasonable estimates. In reality, they might be lower—and in the United States even higher. Third, we assume that the risks of infection are the same nationwide. Fourth, we assume that the incidence of GBS remains the same regardless of vaccine. The lack of vaccine-associated GBS since 1976 suggests that this is not true. Fifth, we assume that the risks of GBS are the same each time the vaccine is given, regardless of the previous number of vaccines received. Evidence suggests the risks may be lower—certainly no higher. Sixth, we assume that everyone over age sixty-five and those of any age with underlying diseases have the same degree of increased risk from influenza. We know that such persons as a group are more likely to die from influenza, but we do not know which members of these groups are more likely to die than other members.

In summary, the risks of flu vaccination are rare adverse

neurological reactions; the benefits are the reduced risks of becoming ill and dying with influenza. The assumptions are too many to devise a precise mathematical risk/benefit ratio, but clearly, based on information now at hand, the benefits of vaccination far outweigh risks for people for whom the vaccine is recommended.

CHAPTER 10

Can You Believe It?

One of the major complications of the subject of influenza is that everyone has a fairly rigid opinion about it—from grandmothers to congressmen, from reporters to physicians. Nevertheless, no matter what you're told, no one is an expert on predicting the behavior of the influenza virus. Those who have studied influenza longer and in greater depth than others have had no end of humbling experiences and fully appreciate the enormous complexity of the problem. There are no simple answers.

During the past few years, much has been said about influenza and influenza vaccines—some of it true, some false. As an example of the prevalent misinformation on influenza, we will examine a sample of the statements made in Washington by our elected representatives, recorded in the *Congressional Record*, House, July 20, 1978, pages H7060-71. The occasion was a debate on funds for the federal government's proposed vaccine assistance program for the medically high-risk groups. We don't attach names to the statements. It is not important who said what; it is important that all of us be aware of the misconceptions about influenza.

1. *Statement:* ". . . in a typical year—mark that: in a typical year—influenza is responsible for 2,000 to 5,000 excess deaths."

Fact: Because the clinical diagnosis of influenza is inexact, we can't be certain how many deaths are caused by influenza annually. However, the impact of an influenza epidemic can be estimated by the number of deaths in excess of that normally expected for that period. In the ten years since 1968 there have been eight epidemics. The estimated number of excess deaths per epidemic year associated with influenza have ranged from a low of nearly 6,000 to a high of nearly 50,000.

2. *Statement:* ". . . a sample of 2,625 people is needed for a reliable test of the safety of the vaccine, but in the clinical study that was undertaken . . . only 834 people participated."

Fact: In the vaccine field trials to which the speaker is referring over 2,000 volunteers participated, not 834. However, at issue here is what the statement "a reliable test of the safety" actually means. To learn if the vaccine will cause an excessive number of sore arms or fever, only a fraction of that number is required. To prove whether or not the vaccine will produce some rare undesirable reaction, such as GBS, 10,000 times that number might be required. It would be impossible to carry out safety tests for all theoretical undesirable vaccine reactions.

3. *Statement:* ". . . CDC's test shows that only one-third of the population receiving at least two flu shots would receive the necessary protection against the flu."

Fact: In the 1978 vaccine trials to which the speaker is referring, 68 to 89 percent of persons twenty-six years of age or older produced protective levels of antibodies to all three viruses in the vaccine after *one* shot. For those under twenty-six, *two* shots were necessary to achieve the same results. Although antibodies in the blood are useful as a measure of vaccine potency, they are only indicative of protection against disease. Actual protection may be higher or lower, depending on many factors.

4. *Statement:* "No satisfactory method has been developed to insure that the vaccine produced by the three or four manufacturers will be similar and will have equal potency."

Fact: Technical problems in laboratory tests of vaccine potency have been legion. Although further improvements in the accuracy of the tests are desirable, current procedures assure the same range of potency for the vaccine produced by each manufacturer, as shown by the results of the 1978 vaccine field trials.

5. *Statement:* "Our experience with the swine flu program tells us that there will be one case of the paralytic disease, Guillain-Barre, resulting from every 100,000 vaccinations, and that in 5 percent of these cases, the person will die."

Fact: No one knows if "there will be" Guillain-Barre. It must be assumed that there *might* be, if all influenza vaccines behave as the swine flu vaccine. GBS occurred in about one out of every 500,000 people over age seventeen who *did not get any* flu shot.

6. *Statement:* ". . . in approximately 100 cases out of 100,000 vaccinations, the recipients will suffer some form of neurologic damage. . . ."

Fact: There is no such evidence.

7. *Statement:* ". . . an additional percentage [of vaccinees] will suffer from hypersensitivity which could accentuate the severity of the flu rather than preventing it."

Fact: This is theoretically possible, but it has never been substantiated and is therefore not known to occur.

8. *Statement:* "HEW claims that some 1,200 deaths

will be prevented by the vaccine should an epidemic break out. In the first place there is no evidence that any such epidemic is in prospect, and second, no substantiation has been provided for the figure of 1,200.''

Fact: "Predictions" can be made only on the basis of previous epidemic patterns. Since nationwide epidemics have occurred in seven of the last ten years, the likelihood of epidemics occurring in any given year is somewhat greater than fifty-fifty. Therefore, to predict an epidemic a year in advance is foolish. It is equally foolish to predict a year in advance that there will *not* be an epidemic. The 1,200 figure cannot be substantiated. It is an estimate, at best.

9. *Statement:* "The cadets at the Naval and Air Force Academies were all vaccinated last year and about 75 percent of them ended up contracting the Russian flu anyway.''

Fact: The statement is correct except for the word "anyway." The vaccine could not have been expected to protect against the Russian flu since that virus appeared after the vaccine was made.

10. *Statement:* "HEW itself admits that there can be antigenic *shifts* between flu seasons, and that a vaccine based on the previous year may not have the proper mix for the upcoming season.''

Fact: True. Antigenic *shifts* occurred in 1957, 1968, and 1977, rendering the current vaccine ineffective. Antigenic *drifts* occur more frequently and may result in *lowered* effectiveness of the vaccine.

11. *Statement:* ". . . in point of fact, the paralysis syndromes that afflicted the swine flu program are found in connection with other flu shots.''

Fact: Studies of vaccine since 1976 have not shown an association greater than that which occurs without the vaccine. But it should be assumed that it might be associated with other flu shots. There is no firm evidence that it will be.

12. *Statement:* ". . . there is one death per 2 million from vaccines. Only one in 2 million. For those who are not vaccinated there are 200 deaths per million from influenza. Actually this shows that immunizations are extremely effective. The ratio is 400 to 1 in favor of immunization."

> *Fact:* This statement uses as its base the excess morbidity figures from a major epidemic year and assumes that immunization would be 100 percent effective if given to the entire population. Such assumptions are risky. First, annual excess deaths from influenza have, since 1968, ranged from zero to over 50,000 and, second, vaccine efficacy has been variable for a variety of reasons. Whether the ratio is 400 to 1 in favor of immunization is anybody's guess. Because persons sixty-five or over and medically high-risk individuals account for the greatest percentage of deaths from influenza, these groups should benefit the most from vaccination. However, we would hesitate to assign a precise numerical value to the benefits of immunization.

13. *Statement:* ". . . approximately 12,000 lives are expected to be saved by this [vaccination] program."

> *Fact:* See statement 8. There the figure was only 1,200.

14. *Statement:* "We have already had this virus circulating in this country last year. People have become sensitized to it and the pattern has been that people were exposed to the virus one year and the second year, whammo, it clobbers you."

> *Fact:* We haven't a clue as to the origin of this statement.

15. *Statement:* ". . . what we really have here is a proposal to market a whole lot of vaccine, unproven as to its effectiveness, against a disease that we do not know will exist."

> *Fact:* Evidence is good that influenza vaccine can

provide significant protection against the disease *if*
the vaccine contains the virus strains that cause the
epidemic. Whether a specific vaccine will confer protection against next year's influenza can never truly
be known until (and unless) an epidemic occurs.

16. *Statement:* "Further, we do not know whether it
[influenza] will respond to the vaccine as a curative or as
an immunizing agent."

Fact: Vaccination is considered a preventive measure, never a curative one.

17. *Statement:* ". . . the administration has requested
to initiate an ongoing annual influenza immunization program. This proposal resulted from the findings of a January 30 [1978] conference, composed of the leading experts
and scientists in the area of public health, influenza, and
immunization practices. Their recommendation, which
has been subject to careful public review, was that high-
risk individuals be immunized on an annual basis against
influenza with federal financial support.

"It is better to be prepared before we have an epidemic.
It may not come, but it may; so this is simply a step in prep-
aration.

"You know, even the vaccine against polio is not 100
percent safe. People take that oral vaccine and you know
what happens? Some of them die from the polio vaccine.
Some of them are crippled, but the benefits far outweigh
the risks. When people know that, it is their judgment
whether they desire to participate."

Fact: Many of you were motivated to read this book in
hopes of getting an answer to the question, "Should I
take the vaccine?" There are no perfectly safe or effective vaccines of any kind. Each vaccine has certain
health benefits. Each vaccine has certain inherent
risks. Society and the individual must make intelligent choices.

APPENDIX 1

Epidemics of Influenza A and B viruses recorded in the United States during the years from 1957 to 1976.

Period of excess mortality	Estimated number of excess deaths due to pneumonia and influenza	Estimated total excess deaths	Type of influenza
Oct. 1957-Mar. 1958	18,500	69,800	A/Japan/57
Mar.-Apr. 1959	1,400	7,900	A/Japan/57
Jan.-Mar. 1960	12,700	38,000	A/Japan/57
Jan.-Mar. 1962	3,500	17,100	B/Maryland/59
Feb.-Mar. 1963	11,500	43,200	A/Japan/62
Feb.-Mar. 1965	2,900	14,900	A/Taiwan/64
Feb.-Apr. 1966	3,700	15,900	A/Taiwan/64
Jan.-Feb. 1968	9,000	23,800	A/Georgia/67
Dec. 1968-Jan. 1969	12,700	33,800	A/Hong Kong/68
Jan.-Feb. 1970	3,500	17,300	A/Hong Kong/68
Jan.-Feb. 1972	5,600	24,600	A/Hong Kong/68
Jan.-Feb. 1973	6,700	24,800	A/England/72
Jan.-Feb. 1976	8,768	26,653	A/Victoria/75

IMPORTANT INFORMATION ABOUT
INFLUENZA AND INFLUENZA VACCINE, 1980-81

Please read this carefully

FLU 7/15/80

WHAT IS INFLUENZA ("FLU")? It is an illness caused by influenza viruses. It generally affects people of all ages. Usually, people with influenza have fever, chills, headache, cough, and muscle aches and may be sick for several days to a week or so. Most people recover fully. A small proportion of cases are particularly severe, and patients may develop pneumonia or other complications. In some past epidemics, about one case out of every thousand was fatal. The risk of complications and death from influenza is highest for people with chronic health problems like diabetes; diseases of the heart, lungs, or kidneys; severe anemia; or chronic illnesses (or medications) which lower the body's resistance to infection. It is also high for older persons generally—particularly those about 65 years old or older.

Influenza viruses frequently undergo changes in their chemical makeup. These changes make it possible to catch influenza even though immunity (antibodies) may have been developed against previous strains of influenza. Thus, having had influenza or influenza vaccine in past years may not prevent getting influenza again.

Although influenza epidemics are unpredictable, some influenza occurs each year. In very large epidemics, as much as 1/3 of the population have become sick and thousands have died.

INFLUENZA VACCINE: Influenza vaccine is composed of killed influenza viruses and is given by injection. The influenza vaccine being manufactured for the fall and winter of 1980-81 offers protection against three influenza strains which recently caused disease in North America (A/Brazil, A/Bangkok, B/Singapore).

DOSAGE: One shot of vaccine should produce protective levels of antibody against the 3 strains of influenza in 70 to 90 percent of adults 28 years of age and older. Persons who are 3 to 27 years of age will need 2 shots about 1 month apart to achieve the same level of protection, unless they received influenza vaccine in the last 2 years. Although there is less information, children 6 to 35 months of age should also get 2 shots. Those who received at least 1 shot of vaccine in the last 2 years, regardless of age, will need only 1 shot this year.

WHO SHOULD GET INFLUENZA VACCINE? Because influenza is usually mild and most people recover fully, routine vaccination of healthy children and adults is not usually emphasized. However, people of any age with the chronic conditions described in the first paragraph, and the elderly, should consider vaccination each year because they are at a greater risk of complications or death if they catch influenza.

POSSIBLE SIDE EFFECTS FROM THE VACCINE: Most people have had no side effects from recent influenza vaccines, although some complained of a sore arm for 2-4 days. Fever, chills, headaches, and muscle aches have occurred in less than 4 percent of recipients. As is true with any vaccine or drug, there is a possibility that allergic or more serious reactions, or even death, could occur. In 1976, about 12 of every 1 million adults who received swine influenza vaccine developed a paralytic condition called the Guillain-Barré Syndrome (GBS) within 10 weeks of vaccination. (Very little information is available on the risk of GBS following influenza vaccination for persons under age 18). GBS also occurred in about 2 out of every 1 million adults who

130

can be expected to recover; 5-10 percent may have some permanent paralysis; and 5-6 percent may die. In 1976, there was an average of 1 death from GBS for every 1.8 million people vaccinated; GBS deaths among vaccinees over age 65 were higher—about 2 for every 1.8 million people vaccinated.

Most information concerning the risk of GBS following influenza vaccination was gathered in 1976. Studies in 1978-79 and 1979-80 did not show an increased risk of GBS in persons who received influenza vaccine. However, it is possible that the risk of GBS which was observed in 1976 may be present for other influenza vaccines. Any risk of GBS should be balanced against the much higher risk of complications (including death) from influenza for the chronically ill and the elderly during influenza epidemics.

Other illnesses, including other neurological illnesses, have been reported among people after they received influenza vaccine, but a relationship between the vaccination and the illness has not been established.

PLEASE KEEP THE UPPER PART OF THE INFORMATION SHEET FOR YOUR RECORDS

TOR BEFORE TAKING INFLUENZA VACCINE:

- Those who have fever or feel ill with something more serious than a cold.
- Those who have received another type of vaccine in the past 14 days.
- Those with allergies to eggs.
- Those with multiple sclerosis, previous attacks of GBS, or other recurring or persistent neurological illnesses.
- Those who are pregnant. NOTE: There are no conclusive data on whether or not the risks from influenza illness or influenza vaccine are the same for pregnant women as for the general population. Because doctors avoid giving any drugs or vaccines in pregnancy without clear need, a doctor should specifically advise a pregnant woman about her need for influenza vaccine.

QUESTIONS: If you have any questions about influenza or influenza vaccination, please ask now or call your doctor or health department before requesting the vaccine.

REACTIONS: If anyone receiving influenza vaccine gets sick and visits a doctor, hospital, or clinic in the 4 weeks after vaccination, please report this to:

I have read the information on this form about influenza and influenza vaccine. I have had a chance to ask questions which were answered to my satisfaction. I believe I understand the benefits and risks of influenza vaccine and request that it be given to me or to the person named below for whom I am authorized to make this request.

INFORMATION ON PERSON TO RECEIVE VACCINE		
Name (Please Print)	Birthdate	Age
Address	County	
State, ZIP		
X_____		
Signature of person to receive vaccine or person authorized to make the request	Date	

FOR CLINIC USE
Clinic Ident.
Date Vaccinated
Manufacturer and Lot No.
Site of Injection
Chronic Disease   Yes ☐   No ☐

FLU 7/15/80

131

Index